How to Heal Yourself

With the Power of Meditation & Chakras

- 2 Books in 1 -

Meditation for Beginners & Chakras for Beginners

Mind, Body, and Spirit Masterclass

© Copyright 2022 - Mind, Body, and Spirit Masterclass -All rights reserved.

The following Book is reproduced below with the goal of providing information that is as accurate and reliable as possible. Regardless, purchasing this Book can be seen as consent to the fact that both the publisher and the author of this book are in no way experts on the topics discussed within and that any recommendations or suggestions that are made herein are for entertainment purposes only. Professionals should be consulted as needed prior to undertaking any of the action endorsed herein.

This declaration is deemed fair and valid by both the American Bar Association and the Committee of Publishers Association and is legally binding throughout the United States.

Furthermore, the transmission, duplication, or reproduction of any of the following work including specific information will be considered an illegal act irrespective of if it is done electronically or in print. This extends to creating a secondary or tertiary copy of the work or a recorded copy and is only allowed with the express written consent from the Publisher. All additional right reserved.

The information in the following pages is broadly considered a truthful and accurate account of facts and as such, any inattention, use, or misuse of the information in question by the reader will render any resulting actions solely under their purview. There are no scenarios in which the publisher or the original author of this work can be in any fashion deemed liable for any hardship or damages that may befall them after undertaking information described herein.

Additionally, the information in the following pages is intended only for informational purposes and should thus be thought of as universal. As befitting its nature, it is presented without assurance regarding its prolonged validity or interim quality. Trademarks that are mentioned are done without written consent and can in no way be considered an endorsement from the trademark holder.

Table of Contents

Foreward 11

Book 1: 15

Meditation for Beginners 15

A Practical Guide to Start Meditating 15

Quiet Your Mind, Reduce Stress and Anxiety, Sleep Better, and Improve Focus with Proven and Time-Tested Guided Meditations 15

Introduction 17

Meditation: What It is and What It Isn't 21

The Main Meditation Techniques 27

Traditional Meditation 28

Intentional Meditation 29

Transcendental Meditation 29

Mindfulness Meditation 30

Walking Meditation 31

Kundalini Meditation 32

Dynamic Meditation 32

Active and Passive Meditation 35

How to Start Meditating 41

Meditation and Routine 51

Where to Meditate and How Long 55

At Home 56

Outdoors 57

Meditation Schools or Specialized Centers 58

Special Locations 60

Breathing and Meditation 65

Ujjayi breathing 68

Kapalabhati Breathing 70

Relaxation Breathing 72

Diaphragmatic Breathing 74

Calming Breathing 76

Breathing for Positivity 77

Alternate Nostril Breathing 81

What Do You Need to Meditate? 85

The 9 Benefits of Meditation 93

Tips for Getting Started with Meditation 101

The 11 Tips for Meditating Better 107

The 13 Most Common Mistakes 115

Step-By-Step Meditations 127

Short Meditation - 1 Minute 128

Short Meditation - 3 Minutes 131

Short Meditation - 5 Minutes 133

Short Meditation for Gratitude - 5 Minutes 135

Short Morning Meditation - 3 Minutes 138

Meditation for Better Sleep - Short - 5 Minutes 140

Meditation to Reduce Anxiety - Short - 5 Minutes 142

Meditation to Reduce Stress - 10 Minutes 145

Mind-Body Connection Meditation - 5 Minutes 148

Meditation to Calm Your Mind - 10 Minutes 150

Conclusion 155

Book 2: 159

Chakras For Beginners 159

A Complete Guide to Balance Your Chakras and Healing Yourself with Yoga, Meditation, Crystals, Essential Oils, and Other Self-Healing Techniques 159

Introduction 161

How Do Chakras Work? 167

The Origin of the Study of Chakras 171

The 7 Main Chakras 173

Root Chakra (1st) 181

Sacral Chakra (2nd) 187

Solar Plexus Chakra (3rd) 191

Heart Chakra (4th) 195

Throat Chakra (5th) 199

Third Eye Chakra (6th) 203

Crown Chakra (7th) 207

How to Balance and Heal Your Chakras 211

Affirmations and Mantras 215

Meditation 225

Yoga 241

Massages 247

Chromotherapy 253

Crystal Therapy 259

Essential Oils Therapy 273

The Power of Chakras: Benefits of Healthy Chakras on Physical, Mental, Emotional, and Spiritual Levels 279

Conclusion 293

Foreword

Self-healing can be done in various ways. The starting point is the understanding that you are a spiritual being in a physical body. Once you are confident with this idea, it becomes clear that to feel truly well you can't only take care of the health of your physical body. To be healthy and to feel good you need to heal your spiritual side too.

Stress, anxiety, panic attacks, sexual disorders, unhappiness, skin rashes, and a lot of other uncomfortable conditions so largely diffused in this modern society, definitely need a medical approach to be healed, but you can help the medical approach and really do the difference in your life by starting to heal your spiritual side.

The first step is to recognize that you have a spiritual side and that this side is just as important as the physical. If you have bought this book, you have already understood this and you are ready to face the next step: how to heal your spiritual side and how to take better care of it.

In the first book of this book bundle, you will discover the power of meditation and the enormous benefits its practice can bring to your life. You will learn to get in touch with your inner self, understand it, and heal it from stress, anxiety, and all other discomforts your inner self may be experiencing.

In the second book of this book bundle, you will discover the energy doors of your spiritual sides. You will understand how the energy that flows through these doors can influence your life and your physical body.

These doors are called Chakras and you will be shown how each of these energy points influences a certain area of your life and can cause you discomforts at a physical level. You will also learn how to heal yourself by healing your chakras through yoga, meditation, crystals, essential oils, and a lot more.

I am sure you will love this trip to the discovery of yourself because it will change your life like night and day. Healing your spiritual side improves your physical health, you will be happier because you feel better, and you will be able to enjoy better relationships, and a wonderful life free from anxiety, stress, anger, and unhappiness.

If you are under medication or you aren't well, please seek medical advice, but use the suggestions in this book to support your medical therapy and make it more effective.

All the information shared in this book bundle has made an enormous change in the quality of my life. My biggest wish and desire is that it will make such a big difference in your life too.

I wish you all the best,

Anja (the author)

Book 1:

Meditation for Beginners

A Practical Guide to Start Meditating

Quiet Your Mind, Reduce Stress and Anxiety, Sleep Better, and Improve Focus with Proven and Time-Tested Guided Meditations

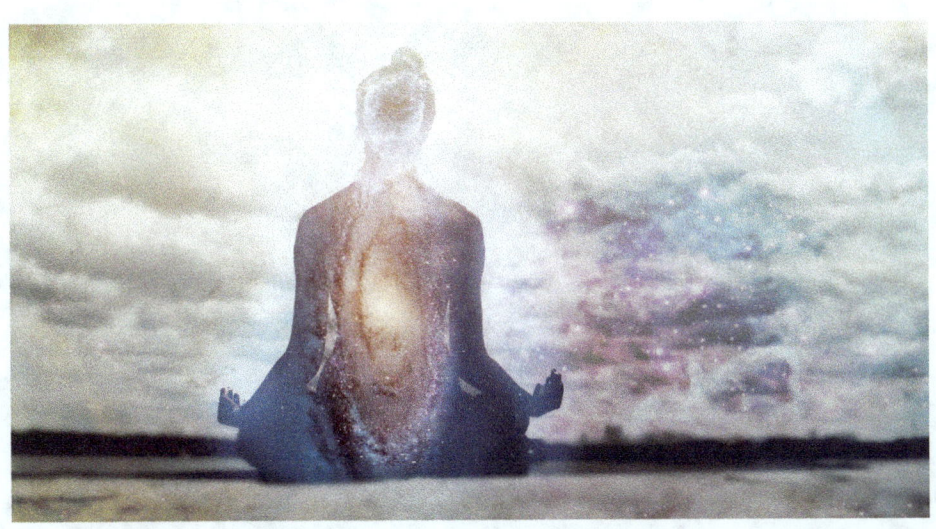

Introduction

Hello and welcome,

I am very happy that you have chosen my book to begin your journey to the discovery of the wonderful world of meditation. My name is Anja and I do coaching and counseling for those who need to rebalance their body, mind, and spirit. I cover topics such as Chakras, Meditation, Yoga, Crystal Therapy, and much more. In addition to my various books, you can find insights on these closely related topics on my Youtube channel, where you can ask me your questions for answers. This is the link to the channel which is called "Mind, Body & Spirit."

https://www.youtube.com/channel/UC5DxslTyhtdH5iQo1UtkO9Q

Now you know a little more about myself, let's get back to meditation. If you have decided to buy this book, you have most likely heard about meditation from many different sources around you, you would probably like to get the fantastic benefits everyone is describing, but you have no idea how to get started. It sounds complicated to you, something that is not in your chords, and that you don't fully understand. Don't worry! You are in the right place.

In this book, you will find everything you need to know to start meditating on your own at home and start enjoying the enormous benefits of meditation in a relatively short time. This is a manual entirely designed for beginners, so you will find detailed information for starting from scratch with the practice. Everything will be explained thoroughly so that it will be understood effortlessly even by those with really zero experience, and it will also be full of tips and suggestions that are always extremely useful when approaching something new for the first time.

You will find some theory in the book, just to do the necessary background such as, for example, understanding what meditation is, what it is really for, and what kinds of benefits it can bring to your life. Otherwise, the information you will find will be practical. In fact, I will explain many things that you will not just read about but will have to apply. I am referring to explanations on how to create your own meditation space, rather than how to breathe, and even complete step-by-step scripts on how to do your first meditations.

As in all other areas of life, it is acting that makes the difference. Action causes a reaction. So, it will not be enough for you to just read the book, if you want the benefits you will have to put the various steps and suggestions into practice. Not only that! You will have to persevere daily and treat meditation as a muscle to be trained. A daily workout, even if only a few minutes long, will bring you incredible results even in a quite short space of time.

Well, I would say that with the premises we are done, so we can set off on our journey to discover the wonderful world of meditation and all its benefits. You are about to discover and experience for yourself why there are so many people talking about this tool that is incredible for well-being, serenity, and happiness.

EVERYONE CAN MEDITATE!

EVERYONE SHOULD MEDITATE!

Meditation: What It is and What It Isn't

The term meditate comes from the ancient Latin word "meditari" which means to think, reflect and study.

By the term meditate, in a broad sense, we mean "to quiet the mind". Meditation is a state of deep peace in which the mind quiets down while still remaining alert.

The main goal of meditation is to bring all our attention right to ourselves to achieve deep inner peace and gain great self-awareness.

Meditation is a very powerful tool, but at the same time, it is very simple to use. To master it in the best way all it takes is perseverance in practicing it, just as I mentioned in the introduction. It will be through practice that you will be able to see the first results. Don't be frightened by this idea of constant practice. You might think that it will take up time you don't have or that you won't be able to integrate it into your daily routine. This is not the case at all.

The daily practice might take up as little as 5 minutes a day, but it would bring huge changes to your life in such a gentle way that it would become part of your routine without you almost noticing it.

Meditating makes us feel good about ourselves, and feeling good about ourselves is a condition that everyone should aspire to, in my opinion. That is why I believe that meditation is a practice suitable for everyone and not reserved for a select few. I also consider it an easy practice because I believe that anyone, with a little practice, can achieve the state of peace and self-awareness required to meditate, regardless of age or life experiences.

The benefits you can achieve by consistently practicing meditation are really many and incredible. It reduces stress levels, brings peace and harmony to the body and mind, strengthens mental and physical health, provides relief from chronic physical pain, improves sleep quality, gives serenity, helps you achieve greater awareness of your body and mind, and also awareness of who we are in our wholeness deep inside ourselves.

Meditation is a doorway to our roots, helping us to root ourselves, anchor ourselves, be present in the "here and now" and be centered.

This does not mean sitting for hours in a certain position, like that of the statue or that of the Buddha. In fact, you might find yourself meditating while doing something else. Maybe you are walking and without even realizing it you might be in a meditative state. It might happen to you when you are in contact with a natural element that you are particularly comfortable with. For example, immerse in the water, while bathing or swimming, you might be in a meditative state. In fact, let's say that the term doing meditation is a bit of a stretch; it would be more correct to say being in meditation, being in a meditative state.

A great many scientific studies have shown how much the mind changes after meditation. During meditation, our brain stops processing information and becomes quiet. Therefore, meditation leads to a deep state of physical and mental stillness. During meditation, the mind is calm and quiet but still alert.

This thoughtless state of peace and awareness cannot come if you concentrate on not thinking. During your first attempts at meditation, you tend to repeat to yourself, "I must not think, I must not think, I must not think!" Tough, you end up having the opposite effect and feeling worse than when you started. This is normal the first few times. That is why it is important not to give up, you have to keep trying and practicing. The state of mindless awareness will come slowly. With constant practice, you will create this state of inner peace, where you stay in touch with the pure essence of what you are in the present moment.

By "what you are in the present moment," I do not mean whether you are male or female, whether your name is Sarah or John, whether you are 20 or 60, whether you are happy, sad, angry, or tired. I am really referring to simply being in that moment, existing, breathing, a simple "I Am," "I Am Here." You are simply a presence in your body. This is meditation.

Meditation is like a muscle and it has to be trained, remember that for every action there is always a reaction, so if you meditate you will always enjoy the benefits. You just need to start with a few minutes a day. One minute, then two, then three, then five... maybe the results won't come right away, but slowly the repetition will change your unconscious mind and that will help you a lot. It will improve your quality of life immensely.

By now you should have understood what meditation is, but, for the avoidance of doubt, let's also see what it is not. All the talk about meditation has ended up distorting many people's ideas, so let's clarify them a bit.

Meditation is not a religious practice, but a practice to get in touch with one's spirituality. Religion and spirituality are two very different things. You are a spiritual being living in a physical body, often the hectic life makes you lose sight of your spirituality, and with meditation you go and get back in touch with it, it puts you back in touch with your spirit, with your spiritual part. Religion, on the other hand, is what binds a person to what they consider divine or sacred. Meditation is indeed used as a practice by many religions, but it is not in itself a religious practice.

Meditation is not a tool to achieve supreme enlightenment. Buddha's story is certainly fascinating and perhaps, with time and a lot of practice, you can achieve deep enlightenment, but there is no guarantee. That is not why you should practice meditation, you should practice it because it makes you feel good. If you set out in search of enlightenment, and you don't see tangible results in that area in a short time, you will give up, depriving yourself of a huge opportunity to live a better life.

In the next few chapters, we will dive into most of the concepts that I have merely mentioned in this first chapter to give you an understanding of what meditation is and how it can change your life for the better.

The Main Meditation Techniques

Many different meditation techniques have developed throughout history in different geographical areas, following different philosophies and traditions. They all are techniques with quite different applications. The advantage is that with so many different techniques, everyone can find the method that suits him best.

In my opinion, all this abundance of techniques ends up creating so much confusion in the heads of beginners, to the point of scaring them off and keeping them away from meditation. So, I would like to provide you with some explanations to easily and quickly clear any confusion you might have.

There are 3 techniques that I think are fundamental and I consider them the main ones for a beginner to start with. The choice of one of the 3 depends on the goal the beginner wants to achieve but also on what is closest to his personality and his way of being. I am referring to traditional meditation, intentional meditation, and transcendental meditation.

I will briefly describe all three so that you can have a clear idea about the main characteristics of each one. At the end of the chapter, I will also mention the other major techniques so that you will be familiar with them, but I recommend further study only when you have become a little more experienced in the practice.

Traditional Meditation

It is also called classical meditation or Zen meditation. To be clear, it is the classic seated meditation, usually cross-legged, that everyone thinks of when meditation is mentioned. The basis of this meditation is breath and stillness. You sit and watch your thoughts go by whilst listening to your breathing. Your mind is focused on the present moment.

The main benefits you get from this meditation technique are:

- Greater self-control

- Excellent observation skills

- Deep self-awareness

This technique helps you eliminate:

- Fear

- Insecurity

Intentional Meditation

Intentional meditation is also called aware meditation or "Vipassana." This term comes from ancient Indian and means "vision" or "looking deeply into things."

It is called intentional because it is based on awareness of our breathing. You practice it by focusing all your attention on an object and its movements. The object can be material or immaterial, that is, it can also be a vision, a visualization.

You focus on a specific image and you do it by nurturing a state of mind. It is intentional and conscious, you practice it to attract a certain result. You focus on a mental demand and a state of mind. The affirmation of what you want is your intention. Your intention is what you have to repeat in your meditation.

The main benefit of this technique is the elevation of your spirituality to a higher level, and from that higher level you can enjoy a new view of life, you gain a much more enlightened view of things.

Transcendental Meditation

Transcendental meditation is practiced by repeating a Mantra, that is, a special phrase or word to be repeated several times during the practice. First of all, it is important to find the Mantra that suits you best, and then it is necessary to recite it with your eyes closed for a certain time during the day. This mantra keeps the mind busy allowing the being to calm down, relax, and achieve inner peace.

The main benefits one gets from this meditation technique are:

- Harmony with our innermost self

- Inner peace

- Tranquility

- Harmony with the world around us

There are, as I mentioned at the beginning of the chapter, so many other meditation techniques. Aside from the three main ones that I recommend you focus on, for the time being, there are four others that, in my opinion, are worth mentioning for your knowledge and, perhaps, for future study when you will become a little more confident with meditation. They are mindfulness meditation, walking meditation, kundalini meditation, and dynamic meditation.

Mindfulness Meditation

This meditation technique is a Western-style revision of intentional meditation. Its practice is based on 3 cornerstones:

1. Focus on the present: here and now

2. Observe without judging

3. Analyze your emotions transparently, without preconceptions

The main benefit of this technique is total acceptance of yourself accompanied by deep self-awareness, which together allows you to free yourself from pain.

The basis of this practice is to be guided by feelings and emotions instead of thoughts. It is considered particularly suitable for those with the need to manage states of anxiety.

Walking Meditation

This practice is performed precisely by walking and its creation is attributed to Buddha himself during his awakening as he walked barefoot across India. As you physically move your body from one place to another by walking, meditation allows you to empty your mind of superfluous thoughts. You arrive, therefore, at your destination with a clearer and more organized mind than when you left.

The main benefits you gain from this meditation technique are:

- Finding peace daily through movement

- Organizing thoughts

- Disciplining the mind

Kundalini Meditation

This meditation technique is a bit more complicated than the others because it takes place in multiple sessions. Each session should awaken the energy of one Chakra and accentuate its benefits. There are seven main Chakras, so we are talking about at least seven sessions. If you are interested in learning more about Chakras, I have written a book about it, easily available in the main online bookstores.

Going back to meditation, kundalini energy is an energy that is spirally twisted at the base of the spine and is released by activating the Chakras.

The benefit of awakening this energy is an immense, very deep joy that flows from the center of your being as a result of full self-realization.

Dynamic Meditation

This technique is part of those techniques called active meditation, just like walking meditation. Its practice requires movement and expression. It is practiced by freeing your deepest emotions and expressing them through the movements of your body. It is possible to do this, for example, through dance (even frenetic dance) using each movement to channel the feelings and emotions that pervade you. As a result of this expression, you can better appreciate silence and calm.

Active and Passive Meditation

In the previous chapter, I covered what you can consider the main meditation techniques. There is another distinction to be made in the area of meditation that I think is very useful to know, even as a beginner, to have a totally clear idea about the various aspects of what it really means to meditate. I am referring to active and passive meditation. I find it important to clarify this point because there is always so much confusion and so many misconceptions about the concept of meditation. Let's see what the difference is and which one is the best option between the two.

We talked in the previous chapter about walking meditation but there are a lot of other examples of active meditation. The first example that comes to my mind is Yoga because I practice it regularly, but for many people, it is the sport they most like to practice that brings them into a meditative state. For some it is running, it is brisk walking by the sea, it is surfing or canoeing or perhaps hiking surrounded by nature.

When you play a sport you love, you enter a flow that generates gamma-type brain waves, which are the waves the brain emits during the meditative state. Very often the sports you love are practiced in contact with nature, and this creates a deep state of contemplation that really puts you in a state very similar to traditional meditation. The state described is only similar tough because traditional meditation is passive. In both cases you are in the flow, you emit gamma waves, you are present in the "here and now", and you are connected to what you are doing. Although these two states have so many similarities, they are actually profoundly different.

Body and mind are deeply linked and connected. So, if the body is doing something like hiking, running, or surfing, that is, it is moving, the mind follows and moves too. When you move your senses are turned outward to pick up the world around it in which you are moving and your mind is in motion to process all the information coming from your senses. In passive meditation, your senses are turned inward to look inside yourself, it is on your inner part that the focus goes.

Having your senses turned outward makes you a victim of the thousands of distractions of the world around you and this prevents you from entering a meditative state in the true sense of the word, that is, a deep meditative state.

The only way you can slow down the mind and reach the deep meditative state is to stop the body from moving. In passive meditation you are still and so the mind can slow down but in active meditation, with the body moving the mind follows, moving in turn.

So, active meditation can definitely work, but it cannot be your only form of meditation if you want to get the typical results of passive meditation. It is certainly better than not meditating completely, but you cannot expect the results that even a few minutes a day of passive meditation can give you.

Active meditation has no precise technique, unlike the various passive forms that have precise techniques on how to sit, how to breathe, eyes closed, attention turned inward, and so on. This is because it is not a true form of meditation, but only a pleasurable state that resembles meditation.

In passive meditation, the senses are turned inward and a state of stillness for the body and mind must be sought. A state of concentration, awareness, and presence in the "here and now." It is the attainment of this state that allows you to enjoy the benefits of meditation, and only passive meditation allows you to reach this state. You reach a totally different state of consciousness and awareness than the one you can achieve with active meditation, which is why the results of the two techniques are not comparable and are very far apart.

Passive meditation allows you to reach a state of pure mindless awareness, a state in which you are alert but deeply relaxed. In this state you are centered, grounded, and rooted. You are in a state of deep relaxation, peace, and harmony that only passive meditation can give you. You cannot reach this state with active meditation because your attention is focused on an outside world full of distractions.

So, I would say that if you have to choose only one form of meditation the best one is passive meditation, where you sit in silence, still, looking inward. Choosing passive meditation is the main point, then you can repeat a mantra to yourself, focus on the breath, an image, or an emotion, whatever form of passive meditation suits you best. It doesn't matter which passive meditation technique you use, the important thing is to achieve a different state of consciousness than usual, a relaxed state of mindless awareness, a state of peace of mind and harmony. Only by reaching the state that passive meditation can give you, you will be able to enjoy the benefits of meditation in your daily life.

If you feel like adding some active meditation to this, it can only do you good, but active meditation alone is not enough to help you achieve the state of well-being that passive meditation can give you.

Do you remember how I concluded the introduction to this book? Everyone can meditate, but most importantly ... EVERYONE SHOULD MEDITATE!

How to Start Meditating

Personally, I have been practicing meditation daily for many years, so most of the tips and advice you will find on these pages have been tested by my own direct experience.

I said before that meditation is a state of concentration, deep listening to self, and presence in the "here and now", whilst being vigilant at the same time. When meditating, we are focused on something, but at the same time, we are relaxed. You might go so far as to say that we are in a "passive" state. As we analyzed in the previous chapter, there are 2 stages of meditation, active and passive, and they are very different from each other. When we feel we are meditating while walking, running, or cooking, we are in a state of active meditation, a meditation in which distractions are involved. In passive meditation, we are sitting, our eyes closed, and focusing exclusively on one thing, turning our senses inward, and not on the outside world as in active meditation. From the detailed description of the dedicated chapter and the brief summary I have given you in the previous lines, you should have understood that you are here to learn passive meditation, the active one will then come on its own according to your time and habits if you wish.

As I mentioned to you earlier, everyone can meditate and everyone who meditates gets enormous benefits. So, don't be discouraged, don't be afraid you won't succeed and don't listen to the skeptics who repeat, "Are you sure you want to do it? No, no! Meditation is not for me!"

So, how do you start meditating?

1. Posture

One of the fundamental aspects of meditation is the way of sitting or meditation posture. I feel like saying that often for those who are just starting out and are absolute beginners, a "perfect" posture is not so fundamental, but there are unavoidable elements of posture that it is best to respect from the beginning.

You must be seated, not necessarily with crossed legs. Your spine needs to be straight, but not rigid.

If you decide to start meditating sitting on the floor with your legs crossed, it is very useful to have a meditation cushion to put under your buttocks so that it supports your back and avoids straining it. You can also use a regular pillow to start with. Over time you will probably prefer to use a meditation pillow (there are many and you will have to choose the one that best suits your needs) for comfort in maintaining your posture. The purpose of the pillow is to make sure that your hips are positioned higher than your knees and that the position is comfortable without straining your back or tiring yourself out. The first few times, you will most likely feel tired anyway, but with time, repetition, and training this will no longer be the case.

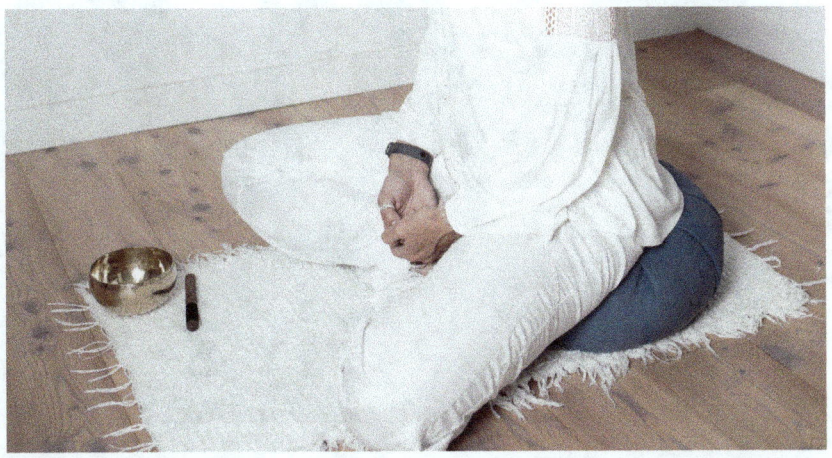

You may also decide to start meditating while sitting on a chair instead of on the floor. In this case, you should sit leaning against the backrest, with your back straight but not stiff, your legs not crossed, and your feet firmly on the ground (rooted). If the backrest does not make you comfortable or does not allow you to sit upright, then do not lean back, sit with your back straight, not stiff, and your legs not crossed, with your feet firmly rooted on the ground.

If, on the other hand, you decide to start meditating sitting on the floor, but on your knees, choose a cushion of those on which you can sit astride so that you still maintain a comfortable position that does not strain your back.

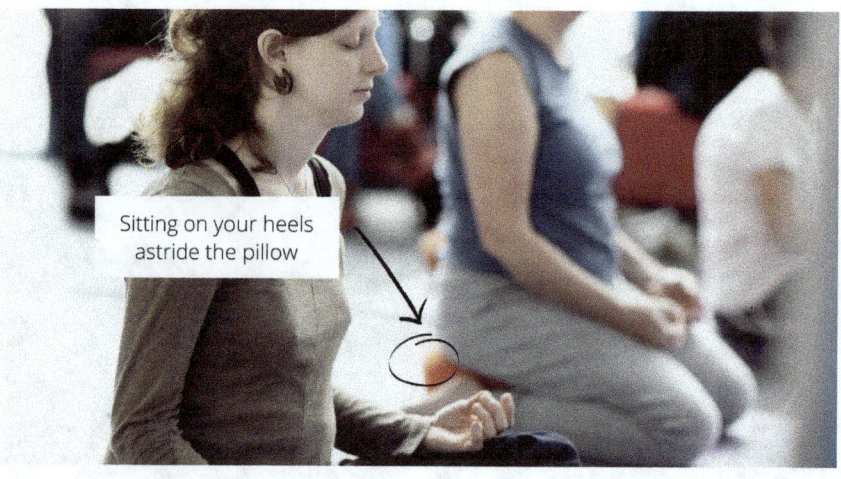

Sitting on your heels astride the pillow

Your hands, in whatever position you choose to sit, rest on your thighs or knees with palms up or down, as you are most comfortable.

2. Close Your Eyes

Close your eyes and take a moment to really begin to immerse yourself in the practice. This is your preparation for meditation. Eliminating visual stimuli will make it easier for you to begin this immersion inside yourself. So, close your eyes and ...

3. Focus

Start focusing on something. There are so many things you can focus on. To get started, I recommend focusing on the most common and simplest one. Starting in the simplest way possible is always the best choice for mastering something new. When you have gained the necessary experience, you can move on to focus on whatever you prefer.

The most common and simple thing to start focusing on is the breath. You have to start by focusing on the flow of your breath, without trying to alter it. You have to let it flow and just observe its flow. You have to concentrate on the breath by observing its flow, visualizing it, and feeling it.

During meditation, some people are better at observing, some people are better at visualizing, some people are better at concentrating on the feelings that arise at the physical level, and some people are better at concentrating on the feelings that arise at an emotional level. For example, focusing on breathing might develop a state of gratitude, rather than one of presence, or joy. When focusing on breathing generates these emotions in you you feel them growing within the body and increasing. These distinctions about what everyone prefers to focus on are actually the different meditation techniques if you remember what we described in the section on the main techniques. For now let's keep it simple, just focus on the breath in the way that is easiest for you.

Surely, when you start concentrating only on your breath at some point different thoughts will start to cross your mind. Don't worry, this is normal, it happens to everyone all the time. It is difficult for people to stay focused only on one image or only on one thing. The mind is like that, we get distracted, other thoughts come across, or physical distractions interrupt our concentration. This causes us to lose the object of our focus, but you don't have to worry because that is part of the practice. What is important is to bring your attention back to the object of your focus as soon as you realize you have lost it. When you notice your distraction it means that you are well along in the process of learning meditation. You have noticed that your mind has left for other shores, that it has started building a movie, but you can come back from there and you can bring your mind where you want, and that is back to the object of your focus.

When you start meditating, especially the very first few times, you will not notice that you have lost your focus, or at any rate, you will notice very few times that the mind has become distracted. In those moments you are not meditating, in truth. With time and practice, you will notice more often the distractions of your mind and you will be quickly capable to go back with your focus to the object of your practice. You will even get to the point where you become less and less distracted throughout your practice and keep your focus and concentration longer and longer.

Well, let's put together the initial suggestions I've given you and create your first little meditation together.

1. Choose your position and sit down.

2. Close your eyes.

3. Take three deep breaths where you inhale through your nose and exhale through your mouth. Use these breaths to create space in your body and mind.

4. After the three deep breaths, you should start breathing only through your nose. The breath should flow easily and freely. Do not control it, do not modify it, just observe it. Observe every time the air comes in and every time the air goes out.

5. Visualize the air entering your nostrils when you inhale and leaving your nostrils when you exhale.

6. It may also help you to feel the sensations in your body, for example, your chest and navel expanding when you inhale and relaxing when you exhale.

7. If a thought comes to distract you, don't worry about it because it is part of meditation. Accept that it has come, let it go, and go back to focusing on the breath. Go back to feeling and listening to your breath.

8. Keep giving your full attention to your breath.

9. If again a distraction or a thought comes, let go. Don't judge yourself for being distracted. Just let go of the thought and bring your attention back to your breath.

10. Stay in meditation for as long as you like. Remember that even a few minutes may be enough at first (maybe 3 minutes or 5 minutes, then you can slowly increase).

11. When you feel ready to return, slowly start moving your fingers on your hands and move them for a few seconds.

12. Now take a deep breath, open your eyes and return to the reality around you.

13. Try to maintain the meditative state for a few seconds even with your eyes open in your surrounding reality so you will bring the positive feelings acquired with meditation into your day. Then get up, but only when you feel ready to do so.

Great! Very well done, you have just successfully completed your first meditation. I am sure it has gone very well. Keep practicing at least once a day and you will see that it will get better and easier every time. In the meantime, proceed with your reading to find out more information, tips, and techniques.

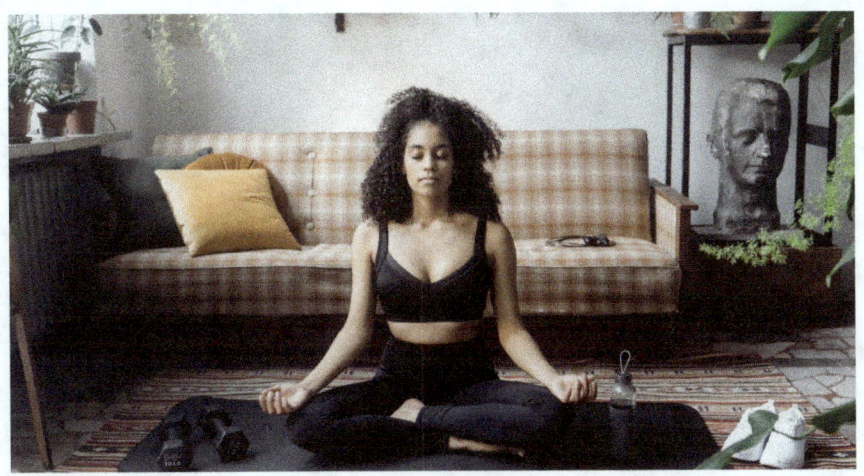

Meditation and Routine

Meditation must become your daily routine. Don't be frightened by my statement because it only takes very little time to achieve enormous benefits. When I say little time, I really mean it. Even a handful of minutes each day can be enough.

Don't imagine that you have to meditate for hours in the perfect lotus position. The important thing is to meditate daily and make meditation part of your daily routine. You don't even have to sit cross-legged on the floor. You can sit in a chair, lie on a cushion or a mat, whatever is best for you, as long as you meditate regularly and consistently for even a few minutes every day.

Nowadays, we all live extremely dynamic, often hectic lives. We are constantly inside our heads, always inside our whirling thoughts, busy doing a thousand things. We are caught up in the lives of other people we are somehow connected to and we interact with them constantly, either directly or perhaps through the various social media, on which we spend a significant amount of time during our days.

For all these reasons, meditation must your daily routine. Amid this chaos and frenzy, it is essential to stop for a moment of calm and peace and to find a moment entirely for yourself.

You need meditation in your routine to have a fixed moment each day in which you are sure to empty your mind and take care of yourself. Not only that, but you also need this moment to recharge your body and mind. Body and mind are deeply connected and to function well they need to be rebalanced, recharged, and reconnected at least once a day. Your daily meditation routine allows you to make all this happen.

You only need a few minutes to close your eyes and try to empty your mind, relax, and try to reach a state of peace. Try to find harmony, a sense of connection, and presence in the "here and now". This is very important, being in the present moment is essential and meditation allows you to achieve this condition.

To be in the present moment you need to turn your attention inward. The world we live in, however, always tries to make you do the opposite. We are always focused on the people around us, on what is going on around us, but not enough on what is going on inside us. Instead, it is so important to regularly take some time to go inside ourselves and be alone with ourselves for a little while.

As I told you, making meditation a small part of your daily routine is very important, but it is equally important to live this experience well. You must not see it as an imposition, nor as a complicated commitment. You must live it simply and lightly, as a small adventure within yourself, a great little journey of your own discovery. A journey within yourself that will bring you so many benefits.

Where to Meditate and How Long

The main purpose of meditation is to be able to concentrate and detach from external stimuli by turning the senses outward. That being said, what is the best place to meditate? The answer is simple and twofold.

The best place to meditate is where YOU can best put yourself in a position to concentrate and turn your senses inward. Having said that, however, I would tell you not to be too conditioned by the place otherwise you risk never meditating. If you get distracted at home, if at the office during your break is no good, you can't every day drop everything and take refuge in a Tibetan monastery to meditate. You have to create an ideal space for yourself where you can meditate daily and then when you can afford it, have a special experience by going to meditate in a special place if you feel the need or dream of having this experience.

Let's look at the main options available to you and the pros and cons of the various environments.

At Home

I would start with your home because it is the most practical place to meditate and the one in which you should feel most comfortable.

The main problem with home arises the moment you share it with someone, be it your family or a roommate. Someone might disturb you during meditation, so it would be ideal to let them know when not to disturb you.

My advice is to create a small meditation corner in your house and make it comfortable. Some small touches can create the atmosphere and facilitate concentration, for example, incense or essential oils, a soft and comfortable rug with your meditation cushion ready for you on it, and comfortable clothes waiting in your corner to wrap you in comfort. In short, there are really so many possibilities, some even with therapeutic purposes, for example, to unblock the Chakras. If this topic interests you, you will find lots of detailed information in my book "Chakras for Beginners," where there is an extensive section on meditation for the Chakras and how to create the ideal meditation corner.

The advantages of this solution are quite obvious. It is a free and practical solution, in fact, you will not have to incur additional expenses, you will not have time constraints, and you will not have to move around to meditate. The disadvantage is the distraction it can represent, both if you live with others who can be a distraction for you, and because the environment itself can distract you by being full of personal stimuli.

Outdoors

There are so many options for meditating outdoors, of course, conditioned by where you live, but let's say there are a few for everyone. Contact with nature helps a lot to get into a meditative state, so this is a very good option, but temperature and weather conditions have to be taken into account.

Let's say that in nice weather or warm weather meditating outdoors is really a worthwhile experience. I suffer a lot from the cold, so for me, this practice is not good if I am in a cold season or place, however it might be good for those who do not suffer from the cold or live in a warm place all year round.

If you live in the city, you can find a space to meditate in a park or public garden. If you live in the country, you could have your own private garden or unearth some other delightful corner in nature. If you live by the sea or in the mountains, you are very lucky. You enjoy the energy of two very powerful elements from which your meditation will benefit enormously, and besides, there will be plenty of quiet and beautiful places to choose from.

Since you need to focus and turn your gaze inward, I recommend that you take 3 elements into account when choosing your temple in nature:

1. Choose a place that is not crowded, so as not to be disturbed and distracted

2. Choose a place that is not a point of transit, for the same reasons

3. Choose a place where it is easy to sit. If you sit on the floor, you need to be able to get up and sit nimbly and comfortably. Otherwise, you might have to opt for a bench, using the position described for chair meditation in the chapter "How to Start Meditating"

Again, the pros are convenience and low cost. If you choose a place close enough to home, the cost of getting there will be very limited and you will not have any particular time constraints. On the other hand, what will constrain you will be the weather, temperatures, and possible intruders to distract you if you have not chosen a secluded enough place.

Meditation Schools or Specialized Centers

This option is more for those who live in cities large enough to accommodate these kinds of facilities, which, although they are spreading widely, are still not available in many of the smaller towns.

In these facilities, it is always possible to avail yourself of a teacher to support you on the path, although, in my opinion, learning to meditate is a very intimate, personal, and individual path that you may want to take alone.

In this circumstance advantages and disadvantages have to be calculated on a more personal level. The possibility of having a teacher for some might be an advantage. Another advantage for some might be that you need an appointment to attend these facilities, and this can help in maintaining a commitment to meditate and regularity in doing so. For those a bit more creative this could, however, be a disadvantage, forcing an act that should be more spontaneous. This submission to schedules would make a spiritual practice that should not be so too mechanical.

Moreover, here it is a matter of adapting to these centers' schedules and not one's own, and this can complicate matters for those whose lifestyles are constrained by rhythms and thighs schedules. Finally, these facilities are fee-based, certainly with options for all budgets, but for many, this can be a drawback.

Special Locations

As I mentioned at the beginning of this chapter, the choice of these special, mystical locations is not about daily meditation. The choice should fall on these special locations when you feel you need a break from daily life when you need to disconnect from your daily routine to immerse yourself in another dimension. The beneficial effect on you is indescribable and it is an experience that I would highly recommend as you begin to gain experience in the practice of meditation.

There are many special locations you can choose from, everywhere around the world, depending on your budget and how far you want to travel.

There are many farmhouses equipped as a place of refuge from everyday life where you can go to meditate. In these facilities, you can immerse yourself in meditation in close contact with wonderful nature as your backdrop.

Other options are monasteries or ashrams. Both of these facilities can be found anywhere in the world, it is up to you to decide whether you want to travel all the way to India or if you prefer one near your city, a choice that also depends on the kind of experience you want to have. I think the concept of a monastery is familiar to pretty much everyone, I mean the place where monks live and pray. The Ashram, on the other hand, is a physical place where you can devote yourself to meditation and prayer, a well-defined place that has this specific purpose. Its name comes from the Indian term "ashrama," which means "place of rest." These are silent places, in close contact with nature, where one goes in search of self through a spiritual path. One meditates, practices the discipline of yoga, studies traditional sacred texts, prays, and travels in search of one's essence through these mystical practices.

The downside of these options, as I mentioned earlier, is that you risk making your meditation practice an occasional factor related to your stay in these facilities. It is self-evident that you cannot attend them daily, and if you only meditate in these places you would find yourself meditating a handful of times a year at best.

If, on the other hand, staying in these facilities becomes an extra to your daily meditation routine, these experiences immediately become a benefit of enormous proportions. They will exponentially improve the quality of your life, accentuating the benefits given by your daily meditation. In addition, the change of experience and setting will help you ensure that meditation remains a spontaneous and deeply spiritual experience, and does not just become a mechanical, forced, and unfelt habit.

Now that we have extensively discussed where to meditate, let's talk about how long you should meditate.

So, "How long should I meditate?" I would say that this question falls into the top 5 that I receive most frequently. The other 4 you can guess because I have answered them in previous chapters. What is meditation? What is it for? How do I start meditating? What technique do I choose? Where do I meditate? For how long?

The answer is, "It depends..."

Let's start with the premise that mediation is an appointment with yourself and must first and foremost be a pleasant time and not an obligation. That is why I say "It depends...," because the right time is the one that gives pleasure to you.

Another consideration we encountered earlier is that it is better to meditate a little, but constantly, than a lot, but sporadically.

Finally, there is the consideration that the depth of meditation matters much more than its duration.

That being said, I reiterate what I said in the chapter on how to start meditating. It only takes a few minutes a day, once or several times a day depending on how you feel, possibly making it a daily appointment, a routine, for you.

You can start with a few minutes the first week (1 to 3 minutes), then increase to 5 minutes the second week. You can choose to do it once a day, at a specific time of the day that suits you best, or several times a day. For example, 5 minutes in the morning to get your day off to a good start, 5 minutes in the afternoon to dissipate stress as it builds up, and 5 minutes in the evening to relax before bedtime.

In subsequent weeks, you might gradually increase to 10 minutes, then 20, then half an hour. Many even go up to an hour. Don't let these time slots make you feel uncomfortable. I reiterate the concept that the right time is the right time for you. However, I can tell you, with deep awareness, that everyone who starts on the path of meditation, as soon as they begin to enjoy the benefits and see the first improvements in their lives, want more, and this brings with it the desire, willingness and desire to extend the meditation time.

So start with a few minutes, try to be consistent, learn to go deep and listen to yourself, meditate for as long as you feel like doing it, and whenever you feel the need for its benefits.

What has been said so far applies to daily meditations. If you go to a monastery or other places of retreat to disconnect from the stress of the world around you, in that case, you have different needs, for longer and deeper meditations probably. Make the most of those experiences to embark on a wonderful journey within yourself.

I would like to end this chapter with a little advice that comes from direct and personal experience. Often during the day, you happen to feel upset because of some events or situations that have happened, other times you feel nervous and insecure about an important event. In all circumstances of discomfort, going for a minute to a quiet corner for a mini-meditation can totally change the fortunes of a day. You really just need a tiny bit of time. Sit down if you can, close your eyes, breathe deeply and consciously, focus your attention on your breath, calm your thoughts and turn to your inner self. That's all it really takes, just a minute or two to eliminate anxiety, stress, insecurity, and other discomforts. You will feel better because of that single minute of meditation, you will be more balanced, calm, centered, focused, and confident.

Breathing and Meditation

Another question I get asked very often is, "What is the right way to breathe during meditation?"

This is a very important question and deserves a detailed answer.

Breathing and meditation are deeply connected to each other. The goal of meditation is to slow down mental activity and we use breathing to achieve this goal. Through breathing, we try to quiet the mind and bring forth inner peace.

The best way to breathe during meditation is to breathe naturally through the nose. Breathing should not be intentionally altered; it should be allowed to flow spontaneously. You must concentrate on the sensation of the air entering and leaving your nostrils and become aware of this process. You have to bring all your attention to this awareness, focus on it, and exclude everything else around you.

As I already mentioned in the chapter on how to start meditating, at first your mind will be crowded with thoughts coming in and making it restless. The more stressed your mind is, the more thoughts will come crowding it as you enter the meditation state. You must let go of these thoughts; you must not follow them even though you will be tempted to do so. You must bring your attention and concentration back to your breath. As soon as your mind wanders off you bring it back to the breath. You will become better and better at doing this through consistent practice.

Remember to keep your breathing natural and fluid, do not alter it, or breathe intentionally. When you breathe naturally, every time you throw out air there is a small pause that is completely natural. It is important not to interrupt this little pause by intentionally altering your breathing because the interruption would cause you to gasp.

The inhalation phase is the phase in which thoughts move and agitate; during the small pause after exhalation, you feel the sense of calmness reverberating in your mind. You must try to take advantage of this calmness to quiet your thoughts before the new inhalation phase. Try to avoid the feeling of numbness that will develop in you during that small pause because that is what makes many people fall asleep when they meditate. Treasure this advice because so many people tell me that they fall asleep when they try to meditate.

There are some meditation techniques with specific purposes where you have to learn to control your breathing consciously. By consciously controlling your breath you can alter your mental patterns, you can calm the mind, make it clearer and more rational to make better decisions, and better manage emotions, especially negative ones. By consciously controlling your breath you can improve sleep quality, concentration level, and memory abilities. Thus, by changing the way you breathe during your meditation, you can change situations and conditions in your daily life. For example, you can better manage emotions, solve insomnia problems, concentration problems, memory problems, and much more.

I would like to share some information that is easy to understand, but a little bit more advanced. For someone, it will be useful for knowledge, while for someone else it will be a useful exercise to take a step forward after the first few weeks of practicing traditional meditation.

In the chapter on meditation techniques, we talked about "Intentional Meditation." Now, I would like to share with you some controlled breathing techniques with specific purposes that you can practice precisely during intentional meditation sessions.

Ujjayi breathing

The term "Ujjayi" comes from Sanskrit and literally means "victory," so Ujjayi breathing is translated as "victorious breath."

It is called this way because its proper practice allows one to calm the mind and be in the "here and now," so this breathing technique "wins" the mind, and controls it by quieting it and making it present. It is the breathing technique performed during yoga and if you are a partitioner you may be familiar with it.

The intentional reasons for its practice during meditation are many and reflect the countless benefits it brings to the quality of our lives. As I have said it calms the mind and gives awareness. In addition, calming the mind reduces stress and nervous tension. By inducing this state of deep relaxation, it is also very helpful against insomnia. It is an excellent tool for deepening the connection between body, mind, and spirit.

How to practice it:

1. Sit in a comfortable position, with your back straight, but not stiff, and your neck and shoulders relaxed. Use a pillow if you sit on the floor. Rest your hands on your thighs or knees. (Go review the chapter "How to start meditating" if you have doubts).

2. Close your eyes, and take three deep breaths inhaling through your nose and exhaling through your mouth. Then breathe in through your nose only and begin to focus on controlling your breathing.

3. Breathing through the nose should be in one smooth, deep flow. Inhalation and exhalation should be the same duration, about 4 seconds each is fine. Count the duration of the first few breaths to gain awareness of the length of inhalation and exhalation.

4. The key part of this technique, however, is that you have to make the temperate of your breath a lot warmer. To do so you must, still keeping your mouth closed and your jaw relaxed, contract the glottis and let the air pass through it producing a sound that resembles an aspirated H. (It resembles the sound you make with your mouth when you breathe on the glass to mist it, but you have to do it with your nose.) The air will make contact with the glottis and the blood vessels will make this air very warm.

5. You will need to hear the sound of your breath throughout the meditation, and you will need to hear it (and thus produce it) on both inhalation and exhalation. Be careful not to close the glottis too much because you

will block the passage of air. The closure should be the minimum necessary to produce the desired sound.

6. Throughout the meditation you should focus on keeping your breathing deliberate, controlled, and steady (4 seconds inhalation and 4 seconds exhalation. You can make 3 seconds and 3 seconds if 4 is too long for you). Go deeper and deeper while maintaining a steady flow and concentration on breath control. Turn all your attention inward with your mind-calming, relaxing, and letting go of all thoughts except breath control.

7. Meditate for as long as you feel. When you decide to stop, bring your breathing back to natural, always from the nose though. Start moving your fingers to slowly return to the world around you, and open your eyes only when you feel ready.

TIP: To tell if you are performing this breathing technique correctly listen to your body. If your chest expands and your abdomen contracts, you are breathing correctly.

Kapalabhati Breathing

The name of this technique comes from Sanskrit and is translated as "Breath of Fire."

It is an energizing breathing technique. With this technique you oxygenate the body and receive three main beneficial effects:

- It improves concentration

- It eliminates feelings of sleepiness and exhaustion

- It fills the body with revitalizing energy

How to practice it:

1. Sit in a comfortable position, with your back straight, but not stiff, and your neck and shoulders relaxed. Use a pillow if you sit on the floor. Rest your hands on your thighs or knees. (Go review the chapter "How to start meditating" if you have doubts).

2. Close your eyes, and take three deep breaths inhaling through your nose and exhaling through your mouth. Then breathe in through your nose only and begin to focus on controlling your breathing.

3. Breathe in as deeply as you can, expanding your abdomen as you do so.

4. Now you must exhale all the air at once, and to do this you must contract your abdominal muscles abruptly and forcefully.

5. Continue with these strong, short breaths and you will begin to feel a warm sensation in the abdominal area. Remember that the abdomen should be relaxed when you inhale and contracted only when you exhale.

6. Meditate for as long as you feel is good for you, although 3 groups of 15 breaths each are recommended for this breathing technique. A full breath is composed of inhalation and exhalation. After 15 full breaths, take a short break and then resume with another cycle of 15 breaths.

7. When you decide to stop, return your breathing to its natural flow, always through the nose though. Start moving your fingers to slowly return to the world around you, and open your eyes only when you feel ready.

Relaxation Breathing

As you can easily deduce from the name, this breathing technique aims to relax and unwind.

The main benefits of this technique are closely related to the state of relaxation in which it places you. Your mind will be free from anxiety and stress, and this condition will also help you sleep better.

How to practice it:

1. Lie down facing up. A gym mat or yoga mat is fine. The important thing is that you are lying on a comfortable surface without anything hurting or bothering you. Extend your arms along your sides with your palms facing upward. If you practice yoga or are familiar with the main postures, this breathing is practiced in the Savasana posture.

2. Get comfortable in the position, close your eyes, and breathe through your nose. Release your mind, focus on your breathing, and on controlling it.

3. Inhale the airflow for 3 seconds and exhale for 6 seconds (you can mentally count to get the rhythm of breathing). Exhaling twice as long as inhaling puts into action the mechanism our body has for relaxing. You should leave a small pause, even just a couple of seconds, between the exhalation and the new inhalation to make the technique even more effective.

4. Meditate and breathe for as long as you need to. Ideally, you should continue until your body and mind are both in a state of total calm, peace, and relaxation.

5. When you decide to stop, bring your breathing back to its natural flow, always from the nose though. Start moving

your fingers to slowly return to the world around you and open your eyes only when you feel ready.

Diaphragmatic Breathing

Its name comes from the part of your body mainly involved in this technique.

Practicing this breathing technique allows you to enter a state of well-being that helps you quickly eliminate stress and is an extremely useful technique for controlling your emotional states.

How to practice it:

1. Lie down facing up. A gym mat or yoga mat is fine. The important thing is that you are lying on a comfortable surface without anything hurting or bothering you. Bend your legs with your feet about 8 inches apart. Place one hand with the palm on your chest and one hand with the palm on your belly. The hands allow you to feel your diaphragm.

2. Get comfortable in the position, close your eyes, and breathe through your nose. Release the mind, focus on your breathing, and on controlling it.

3. Bring your attention to your belly. Breathe in deeply through your nose and let the air go into your belly. Then slowly exhale. It would be ideal to exhale through your nose. If at first attempts, you just can't do it, you can exhale through your mouth, but your goal should be to complete the whole breath properly through the nose. Exhale naturally, without forcing the air out. The purpose of the hand on your chest is to make sure that this does not rise. Instead, you need to feel the belly rise and the hand resting on it will allow you to do this.

4. Meditate and breathe for as long as you feel necessary. When you decide to stop, bring your breathing back to its natural flow, always from the nose though. Start moving the fingers of your hands to slowly return to the world around you and open your eyes only when you feel ready.

TIP: To tell if you are practicing correctly you should have the hand on your chest completely still both when you inhale and when you exhale. The one on your belly, on the other hand, should move and follow the movement of your breath by rising and falling. If the hand on your chest rises, it means you are not using your diaphragm to breathe and you need to try again and practice.

Calming Breathing

Some call this technique the "4 7 8 Breathing". The first name comes from the state it allows you to reach, while the second comes from the breathing times to practice it, which I will explain in a moment.

How to practice it:

1. Sit in a comfortable position, with your back straight, but not stiff, and your neck and shoulders relaxed. Use a pillow if you sit on the floor. Rest your hands on your thighs or knees. (Go review the chapter "How to start meditating" if you have doubts).

2. Close your eyes, and take three deep breaths inhaling through your nose and exhaling through your mouth. Then breathe in through your nose only and start focusing on controlling your breathing.

3. Breathe in for 4 seconds. Hold your breath for 7 seconds. Exhale for 8 seconds. Repeat the cycle.

4. Meditate and breathe for as long as you feel necessary. When you decide to stop, return your breathing to its natural flow, always through the nose though. Start moving your fingers to slowly return to the world around you and open your eyes only when you feel ready.

Breathing for Positivity

Some call this technique the "3 5 3 Breathing". The first name comes from what it enables you to achieve and the second from the breathing times to practice it, which I will explain in a moment.

The main purpose of this technique is to expel all negative energies from the body to remain pervaded by positive ones. As the oxygen circulates, it will cleanse your energy, eliminating anxiety and negativity, and leaving you present, centered, and focused.

How to practice it:

1. Sit in a comfortable position, with your back straight, but not stiff, and your neck and shoulders relaxed. Use a pillow if you sit on the floor. Rest your hands on your thighs or knees. (Go review the chapter "How to start meditating" if you have doubts).

2. Close your eyes, and take three deep breaths inhaling through your nose and exhaling through your mouth. Then breathe in through your nose only and start focusing on controlling your breathing.

3. Breathe in for 3 seconds. Hold your breath for 5 seconds. Exhale for 3 seconds. Repeat the cycle.

4. Meditate and breathe for as long as you feel necessary. When you decide to stop, return your breathing to its natural flow, always through the nose though. Start moving your fingers to slowly return to the world around you and open your eyes only when you feel ready.

Before I conclude the chapter on breathing there are a couple of points I would like to bring to your attention. First, you may have noticed that throughout this section, and in the book in general, I always emphasize that you have to breathe through your nose. This is not accidental. On the contrary, it is not only important but fundamental.

Only by breathing through the nose can our body control the perfect and optimal intake of CO_2 and release NO, which strengthens the immune system, stimulates blood circulation, and helps sexuality. When you breathe through your mouth you expel too much CO_2.

When air passes through the nostrils it is filtered of impurities and is, therefore, of better quality than air inhaled through the mouth, which does not have this filtering function. The nose also warms the air and humidifies it before it enters our internal organs. The mouth cannot perform these two functions either. Therefore, when you breathe through your mouth, you are putting too dry air into your organs and, often, that air is also too cold compared to the ideal temperature of that organ, which will consume your energy to bring the air temperature up to its ideal standard.

Breathing well and consciously can therefore bring so many benefits to your well-being, not only on a physical level.

Our breathing influences our emotional state too and, on the other hand, our emotional state controls our breathing. This is why breathing well and knowing how to control your breathing are so important for your well-being. If you are breathing laboredly, you will find yourself in a state of anxiety and stress. If you are anxious and stressed your breathing will be quite labored. I am sure you have noticed it before.

So, I recommend analyzing your breathing, just because breathing is natural does not mean you are doing it correctly. Throughout your life, you may have picked up bad breathing habits without even realizing it. Use what you have learned in this chapter to do a little analysis. Then use meditation to practice a better kind of breathing. Slowly start using the techniques you have learned to improve the way you breathe throughout your day. You will gain huge benefits by simply breathing better during your day.

You may have noticed that in the chapter on "How to Start Meditating" in step 3 (and also in this chapter) I wrote about taking 3 deep breaths, inhaling through the nose, and exhaling through the mouth. This is one of the rare cases where I recommend mouth breathing, but there is a reason. Exhaling through the mouth is very useful in times of anxiety, stress, and nervousness because it helps release the tension that pervades you. I find it a useful practice for beginners in meditation because they are often a bit tense from facing something new and many times they have accumulated and never discharged tensions that complicate their first approaches to the new practice.

Another circumstance that I frequently notice in those who have never meditated or approached disciplines such as yoga and some martial arts is that they breathe mostly through their mouths and approaching breathing only through their noses seems difficult for them, almost as if they are not getting enough air into their bodies. The way they breathe is mainly a habit, I have already explained why nasal breathing is the most correct. I would like to give a few small suggestions to override the habit of mouth breathing and start breathing mainly through the nose, in case you are part of this group of people.

First, throughout the day try to keep your mouth closed as much as possible, this will somehow prompt you to make more use of your nose. There are several nasal breathing exercises. I feel like recommending one in particular to you, both to strengthen the use of the nose in breathing and to make sure that the nostrils are free and always working at their best.

Alternate Nostril Breathing

When we breathe through our nose to us it seems that we are always using both nostrils, but in fact, we are not. It is a completely natural process; our body chooses to use only one nostril rather than another. It usually chooses to use for breathing the one opposite the half of the brain that is doing most of the work at that given moment.

The benefits this exercise brings are many. As mentioned earlier, it allows the nostrils to be kept wide open at all times, if practiced regularly. It also creates a profound balance between mind and body and is therefore great for keeping nervousness away and staving off the onset of anxiety.

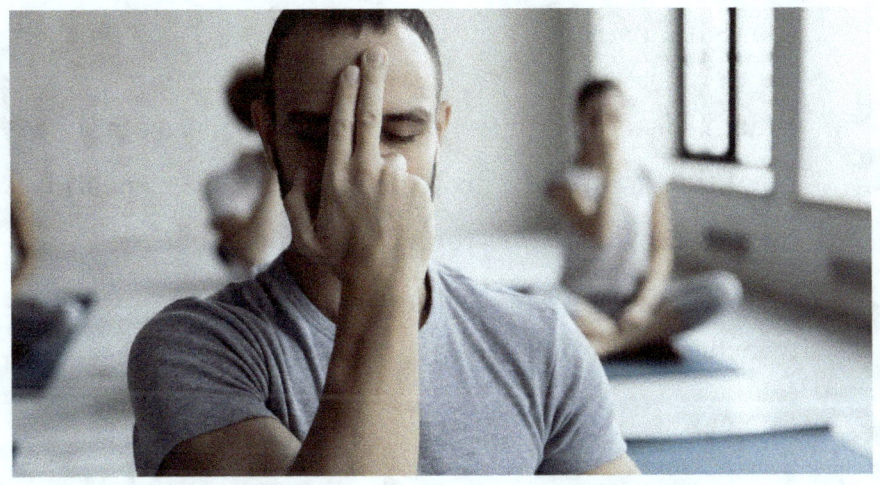

How to practice it:

1. Sit in a comfortable position, with your back straight, but not stiff, and your neck and shoulders relaxed. Use a pillow if you sit on the floor. Rest your right hand on your thigh or knee. Rest the index and middle fingers of your left hand in the space between your eyebrows.

2. With your thumb close the left nostril. Exhale the air already foraged through the right nostril and then inhale again through the right nostril.

3. Remove thumb pressure and clear the left nostril and close the right nostril with the ring finger and little finger. Exhale through the left nostril and then inhale again through the left nostril.

4. Move your fingers as described above and exhale from the right nostril.

5. What is described in the previous points is a complete breathing cycle with this technique. Practice repeating the cycle several times for a few minutes, 15 times is a good repetition time. Remember to complete the exercise by exhaling through the right nostril.

Well done! You now have a great deal of useful information about breathing. All you have to do is put it into practice in conjunction with your meditation sessions to enjoy the immense benefits that both practices can bring to your life.

What Do You Need to Meditate?

I am often asked if anything, in particular, is needed to meditate. No, you do not need anything special to meditate; in fact, you can meditate by simply sitting in a chair.

However, various gadgets can make your meditation more comfortable, especially if you decide to meditate sitting on the floor in the classic meditation position (which is called Sukhasana, meaning "comfortable position").

1. The Mat

The first thing that comes to my mind is the mat. I am referring to gym mats, those commonly used for doing yoga are a perfect solution. They give some comfort and softness. If you meditate outdoors they prevent you from getting dirty, feeling the dampness off the ground and its eventual roughness.

This is especially true for beginners. With time you may begin to appreciate meditating outdoors in direct contact with the earth. It is a wonderful experience feeling the Earth's energy flowing directly into you, without interference. Feeling the warm sand beneath you, the earth between the roots of a tree, or the grass of a meadow is great, but for those who are just starting out it is a bit uncomfortable because you are not yet trained or used to it, so you might find a mat useful at least at the beginning.

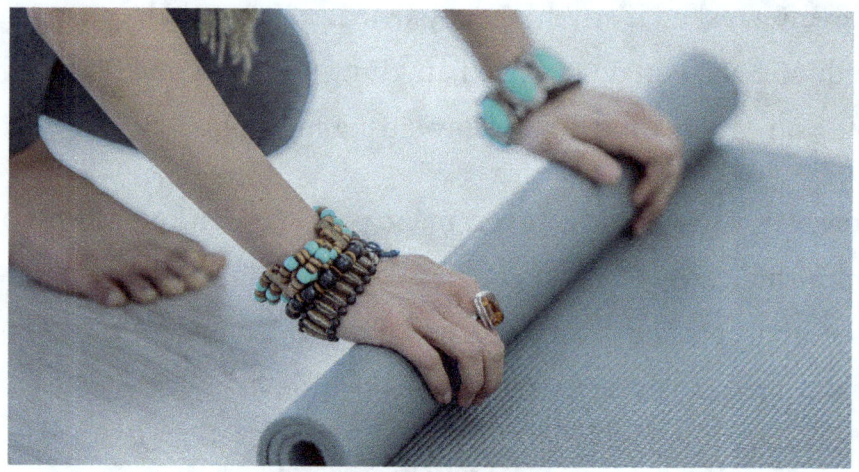

2. Meditation Pillows

You can find them in many shapes, materials, and sizes. They all have the same function of making you feel comfortable during your meditation. I mentioned their use in the chapter on "How to start meditating", and to choose the most appropriate one, you need to figure out what position you are most comfortable sitting in.

Especially in the beginning, using a cushion is always recommended. Your body is not yet trained and accustomed to holding the Sukhasana position or even sitting with your back straight for too long. Therefore, without the help of a cushion, your back may hurt, or the part you are sitting on may be sore because the mat is not thick enough. Conditions of pain or lack of comfort would put your body in such a tense state that it would become an obstacle making your practice more difficult to perform, which is why you might need a good cushion to start with. Over time you may no longer feel the need for it, although this certainly depends a lot on age and physical condition.

Of course, you can also use a pillow you already have, perhaps folding it up or otherwise adapting it to your need.

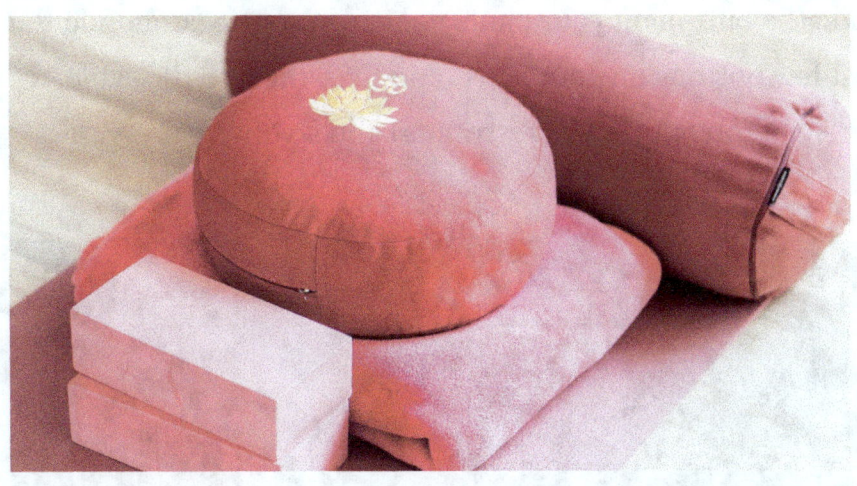

3. Comfortable Clothing

Practicing wearing soft clothing that does not compress and oppress you is a huge benefit to your practice because it is easier to relax while wearing comfortable clothing.

If you meditate indoors you can certainly equip yourself with whatever makes you feel most comfortable, if you meditate outdoors you might consider an outfit that is comfortable but does not make you feel uneasy if you were to meet other people.

If you meditate in the office, you don't need to change, but it might be very helpful to take off your jacket, loosen your belt, undo the button on your pants, take off your tie, and undo the first few buttons on your shirt (and for ladies it's the same, try to get rid of too oppressive restraints) and so on.

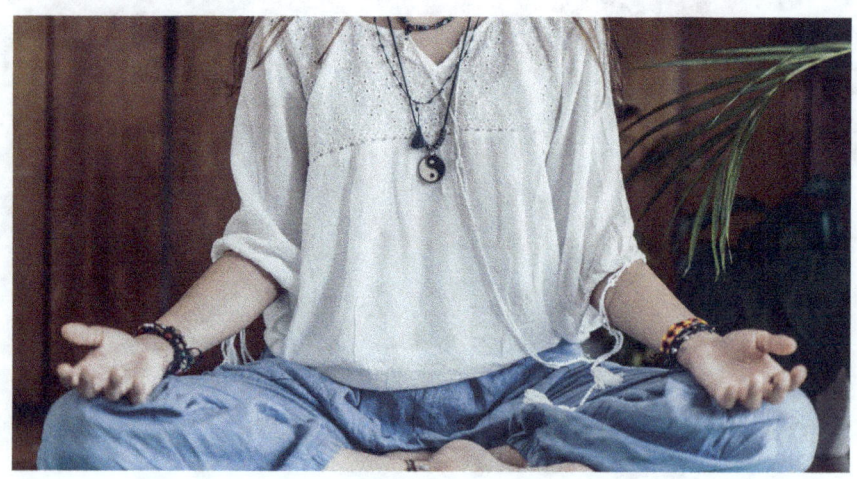

4. Furnishing

This covers a more advanced stage, but it is worth mentioning. If meditation becomes an integral part of your life, as I firmly believe it will, at some point you will feel the need to carve out a little corner of your home that will become your own little sanctuary, your own meditation corner.

You will certainly want to furnish it in some way and decorate it so that it will be even more personal, so that it will be pervaded with energy, and you will just walk into it to feel better and leave out all the ugliness of your day. I'll tell you a little bit about mine to give you an idea, and if you want to go deeper, as I already told you, in my book "Chakras for Beginners" you can find a lot of useful information. I put soft mats on the floor with the colors of the Chakra energy. I scattered the mats with colorful pillows, again to encourage the energy. I added a very low wooden coffee table on which there is an incense burner in which I burn different incense according to the energy I want to stimulate, stones and crystals for all 7 Chakras also lay on that table so that they pervade my energy corner, and last there is a small speaker that I use to broadcast the sounds of nature or to play relaxing music or guided meditations.

Lighting is also very important. In this case, there are mainly three options. You could choose an adjustable intensity lamp placed in a corner and set it to a different intensity according to your needs. You could use candles to set the mood. Finally, you could opt for a Himalayan salt lamp that gives off a warm, soft light with a strong emotional impact. Here the choice is really yours. I can tell you that I do some of my mentor's guided meditations in total darkness, wearing an airplane mask to cover any source of light, but in most cases, I prefer a soft light with warm tones.

In your corner, you might want to put curtains, and sofa covers, you might prefer an essential oil diffuser instead of incense, and you might choose a salt lamp rather than candles. The important thing is that the place reflects your personality and your taste, makes you feel good and gives you the energies and the emotions you need.

Many people find it unnecessary to create this corner because they prefer to meditate outdoors, and the impact of nature infuses them with the same energy. I have found it essential because living in a big northern city, the weather has often been a hindrance, as has contact with nature, which can be reached in rather long spaces of time if you are not lucky enough to live near a decent park to go and practice in. So, consider investing some time and a little money in creating your own little corner of the world. If you are also as creative as I am, you will find it an enjoyable, fun, and ever-evolving activity. Your space will evolve with you, reflect your changes, and always make you feel good.

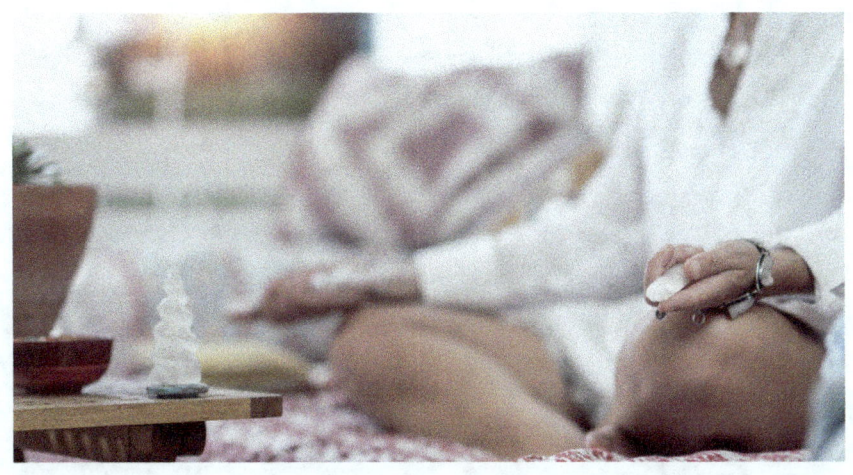

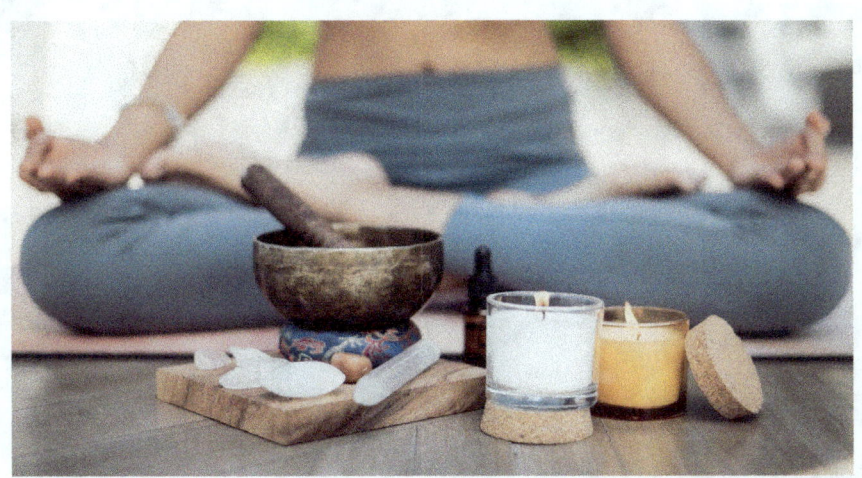

The 9 Benefits of Meditation

The benefits of meditation are measured through the positive changes that occur in your daily life. The happier you feel and the more you feel in control of your life, the more effect meditation is having on your daily life.

The purpose of meditation is to make you a better version of yourself and it does this by helping you to eliminate old, narrow mental patterns and limiting habits. With constant meditation, you will create habits and mental patterns that are much more positive and functional for living a wonderful life. You will gradually see this wonder unfold like a small miracle in all aspects of your life.

Meditation allows you to feel better mentally and emotionally, and this has a huge reflection on your physical well-being. If you are well emotionally and mentally, these two factors will not weigh on the health of your body and you will feel better in general. It is easier to get sick for those people who have emotional or mental problems and, in fact, this category of people is always plagued by a thousand aches and pains. Meditation can help you get out of this loop.

Let's see together what are the main benefits that each of us can gain by consistently meditating for at least a few minutes a day.

1. Meditation Reduces Stress

Many medical studies have shown that meditation is an excellent tool for reducing symptoms given by stress.

Stress is given by the increase in our bodies of cortisol, a hormone that is also commonly referred to as "the stress hormone." When levels of this hormone in our bodies rise we feel stressed mentally and physically. Cortisol creates the release of inflammatory substances that have a whole range of repercussions on our bodies.

Stress tends to create states of anxiety and depression, deteriorates the quality of sleep, causes fatigue, makes your thinking lose clarity, and can cause high blood pressure.

Being able to reduce stress through the practice of meditation can bring enormous benefits to the practitioner's life, reducing the risk of incurring all these uncomfortable states.

2. Meditation Helps Control Anxiety

There are an increasing number of medical studies conducted on people who regularly practice meditation that prove the deep benefits you can gain.

Numerous studies have shown that those who regularly practice meditation tend not to be plagued by anxiety or, at any rate, can control it much better and not be overwhelmed by it.

Meditation is, in fact, a very useful exercise to combine with the various medical therapies given by doctors to patients to manage social anxiety or panic attacks.

If you work in a very competitive environment it can help you relieve the anxiety and stress of everyday situations.

By reducing anxiety, you also reduce the possibility of becoming involved in diseases that arise from anxiety and its various side effects.

3. Meditation Helps Manage Emotions

Meditation can be used to create emotions and feelings other than those we experience. If you are plagued by negative feelings and emotions, which tend to make you feel depressed, meditation allows you to create positive feelings. With these new positive feelings you can, then, create a more positive overall outlook and positive habits, to live life more peacefully. You also learn, in this way, how to deal with painful events and live at peace with yourself and the world.

4. Meditation Gives You Awareness

As I mentioned in the introductory part of this chapter, meditation allows you to become the best version of yourself.

As you get to know yourself better and on a deeper and more intimate level, you become more aware of yourself. This awareness leads you to be better with yourself, but also to relate better to others and to the world around you. You will be better off in your life because you will have healthier relationships with those around you, and with yourself, and solving problems will become easier.

Through meditation, you will be able to identify harmful thoughts and bad, weakening thought habits. Only by knowing these negative points, can you take action on them and turn them into positives.

5. Meditation Makes You More Mindful

When you meditate and bring all your attention to the breath, mantras, sensations, emotions, or whatever the object of your meditation is, and you learn over time to keep this attention longer and longer, you generate tremendous benefit in your daily life as well.

This ability that you learn and improve during meditation to maintain attention for longer and longer times also occurs in your daily life.

Several scientific tests have been done on this benefit, from which it was found that those who practice meditation on a sustained and consistent basis can maintain attention at high levels for longer, without getting tired even in stressful situations, than those who do not practice meditation. The test was done in highly competitive work environments and those who meditated managed to stay focused and undistracted for longer times than their colleagues who did not practice the discipline.

It emerged from this test that repeated practice of meditation reverses patterns of brain functioning that cause a lack of attention and the mind's tendency to wander, thus leading those patterns to work based on attention and focus.

This also leads to a decrease in worries because the brain is focused on what you choose and not wandering around getting lost in creating negative scenarios that will probably never come true, as often happens to those whose minds have a great tendency to wander. You exercise healthy control over your thought patterns and learn to redirect your thoughts positively.

6. Meditation Improves Your Memory

Because of the important improvement in attention that meditation gives you, you also gain a strong mental clarity that exerts a beneficial effect on the quality of your memory.

A clearer mind helps you remember things better. It also helps you keep your mind younger, preventing the effects of aging from occurring too soon and, in many cases, delaying them.

7. Meditation Makes You Sleep Better

As I mentioned in the conclusion of the fifth benefit, through meditation you learn to redirect your thoughts, thus moving the mind away from negative ones and toward positive ones.

Often insomnia, or at any rate poor sleep quality, is attributable to the thoughts we allow to haunt our minds. By being able to redirect these harmful thoughts you will be able to improve sleep quality.

According to scientific experiments on sleep quality, those who meditate fall asleep earlier and sleep longer and deeper.

However, it is not just a matter of thoughts. When you meditate you learn to let go of tension and relax your body and mind. These skills are very useful to fall asleep faster, and the sense of peace that accompanies meditation makes you sleep better and longer.

8. Meditation Makes you Become Kinder

As mentioned in several of the benefits listed in this chapter, meditation helps you positively redirect your thoughts. It also allows you to go very deep within yourself. In this way, you can generate deep, positive feelings toward yourself and then expand them to other people in your world.

You develop love and kindness toward yourself, and you can also share these feelings with those around you. This helps you feel more comfortable in a social group, not feel anxiety from contact with others, and manage anger better. The combination of these benefits helps you deal with difficult relationships with your partner, conflict marriages, or complicated family situations because you develop empathy, positivity, love, and kindness.

9. Meditation Helps You Fight Bad Habits

Daily behaviors and actions are 95% dictated by your habits. Often, you fail to achieve your goals in life because you have some bad habits that hinder you. Changing habits is a process that requires hard work, which is well rewarded by the benefits you gain. However, meditation tends to make this process much easier.

First, meditation helps you develop self-control and self-awareness, which are key elements in changing your habits for the better. Then, through meditation, you can direct impulses, emotions, and attention where you want, being able to understand why you behave in a certain way. In this way, you develop the willpower to correct that wrong habit that is hindering your success in any field.

The examples of hindering habits are so many and in so many areas. Think of someone who is looking for love but cannot stay faithful. Think about someone who wants a fabulous body but can't quench the nervous hunger. Think about someone who wants to have more money but spends more than he earns each month. Really, meditation can bring improvement and well-being in all areas of your life, at the cost of a handful of daily minutes that you can take away from useless activities, like watching TV.

Tips for Getting Started with Meditation

Start with a little. When you want to turn a practice into a habit, you have to start with little, but consistently, every day. Don't start with half an hour, but with a maximum of 5 or 10 minutes, possibly every day, as often as possible anyway.

Make it easy. Don't try a thousand meditation techniques, a hundred apps on your smartphone, and listen to ten different teachers. That would certainly complicate things for you. Try maybe two or three techniques, select a couple of apps to try, or pick a master or two to follow. Then figure out which technique you feel most comfortable with and focus on that. I recommend picking one or two at most to start with.

Schedule your meditation. Decide on a time and, if necessary, set the reminder via an alarm clock on your smartphone so you don't forget. It will seem a bit forced and lacking spontaneity at first, but it is not easy to develop new habits and you need to take advantage of all the tools you can to do so. Of course, on the other hand, you should not experience it as an unpleasant obligation. When the phone rings you should not be annoyed at the reminder but happy that it is time to meditate, a time to devote to yourself and your well-being. The purpose of scheduling meditation is to make the appointment with yourself as welcome and natural a habit as eating, showering, or dressing. You always find time to eat, shower, or dress in the morning. Similarly, it will have to be for meditation, another of the basic and indispensable elements for the well-being of your life.

Keep realistic expectations. You are a lot of conversations around you about meditation, and with all this talk you end up setting unrealistic expectations. Many people expect to receive enlightenment as soon as they start practicing. The first benefit you will get is to feel well, which seems to be an incredible accomplishment in a society where stress, anxiety, and emotional distress are always around the corner waiting for us. So, think about those realistic expectations when you decide to start to meditate. First of all the expectation of feeling well and continuing to get better and better. With time and practice, there will also be room for great revelations.

By meditating with the idea of doing good for yourself and experiencing meditation as taking time just for yourself, you will begin to make a very deep connection with yourself and begin to see the first immediate results in your outer world. You will begin to react differently to situations and circumstances, and you will relate differently to people in your personal life, but also in your professional life. You will feel calmer, more relaxed, and with a much clearer mind.

Give yourself a goal and a reason. Set a small challenge for yourself and win it! Set a precise number of days during which you will meditate and then find the motivation to do it. You can find the motivation by analyzing why you decided to start meditating, that is your why. For example, a good challenge might be to meditate 5 minutes a day for 21 days in the evening, if your reason for starting is to improve sleep quality or avoid insomnia. You have a very good reason to achieve your goal, and you will bring home a great victory. By the way, 5 minutes a day for 21 days is a good goal, it's a good challenge to yourself, absolutely within your reach. You might consider starting here if it doesn't seem too overwhelming. I can assure you that with a good why you can do it with no problem.

Don't judge yourself. Try to treat yourself as kindly as possible. Many people get angry and resent themselves if they make mistakes while learning to meditate. If while meditating, you find you are chasing a thought, don't get angry with yourself, just let it go and bring your attention back to the object of your meditation. You have to let go, accept whatever is happening, accept yourself, embrace yourself, and embrace the moment. Don't get nervous, just accept what comes, and be with yourself. I know it can be difficult and frustrating because you feel like you're doing it wrong or you're not really meditating, but that's okay, let go, forgive yourself, and keep trying. With time and practice, you will continue to improve and stay well focused on your meditation, you soon won't find yourself getting distracted anymore, or chasing random thoughts.

<u>Try guided meditations for initial help.</u> In this book, you will find a chapter with step-by-step transcriptions of 10 guided meditations. You will also find transcriptions of guided meditations in the chapter on "How to start meditating" and in the chapter on "Breathing and Meditation". On my YouTube channel, you will find audio versions of some of them, and as we said before, online you can find many such apps and resources. You can try them to see if they help you, at least in the beginning. If you get distracted while trying, remember the previous point, don't get upset, and keep trying. I personally, when I first started, preferred those that in an introduction explained what to do and then left background music where I could proceed in intimacy to do what was described in the introduction. In other guided meditations, the teacher guides you throughout the process. The preference for one or the other guided meditation is subjective. It is such an intimate practice that some people prefer to do the whole process alone and without guidance, which is why I left this suggestion for last. That is also why I have included step-by-step texts, to give you a

reliable and complete guide, without having to resort to guided audios, if the procedure is not for you.

The 11 Tips for Meditating Better

1. Choose the Best Time

Morning is a good time to meditate because we have just gotten up and the mind is still quite free, not clogged with all the thoughts and information that usually crowd it throughout the day. In addition, meditating in the morning allows you to carry the benefits of the practice with you throughout the day.

If you need to improve the quality of your sleep you might find it more helpful to meditate in the evening.

If, on the other hand, work stresses you out, it might be helpful to take a meditation break during the workday to find a moment to disconnect and relieve stress.

2. Choose the Best Place

It is important you meditate in a place where you feel comfortable otherwise you will find it very difficult to immerse yourself in the meditative state. It is also useful to find a quiet and peaceful place (even if you meditate in the office, I'm pretty sure you can find such a place).

When you start to become a little more experienced, to train your concentration you may want to choose a place that is not completely silent but has some noise, to train you to maintain your concentration despite this distraction.

3. Be prepared

Before you begin your practice I recommend that you drink if you are thirsty or pee if you need to. This is to prevent these circumstances from disturbing your concentration. Especially in the beginning, the fewer distractions you have, the easier it will be to get into the practice.

Clothing is also part of the preparation phase. Meditating in clothes that are comfortable and possibly made of natural fibers helps you feel more comfortable. If you meditate, for example, in the office and are wearing something constricting, loosen one or more buttons, and undo your belt or tie, so that you are relaxed and not constricted.

Don't forget your posture while getting ready. It should be comfortable and allow you to keep your back straight when you sit down. Whether on the floor or in a chair, prepare your seat with cushions appropriate for your comfort.

4. Find Your Why

Having a why when you meditate is useful for a variety of reasons. First of all, as I said in the previous chapter, it is useful because it keeps you consistent in your practice, and consistency is essential to achieve results in meditation (as in any other discipline you undertake).

Second, it is very useful for choosing your mantras, intentionalities, or what you decide to focus your meditation on. So, find your motivation, find the reason why you decided to start meditating.

5. Stop

In a fast-paced world like the one we live in, the concept of stopping may seem a bit strange and impossible. However, you need it to feel good. You also need it to meditate better.

You need to try to stop the avalanche of information that the world around you tries to send to your brain every second. Try to stop your thoughts during the day and pay attention to what you are doing. It will come in handy during meditation.

When you walk to the bus stop after work, turn off your phone, put it in your bag, and try to walk without thinking about anything in particular. While you are cleaning, put your usual gestures into motion without thinking about anything in particular. These little breaks given to your mind will help you meditate better, and you will also feel the benefit throughout the day. They are a bit like active little meditations, like when you practice yoga or run. Take a break from the hustle and bustle of the world and try to be present in the "here and now."

6. Remember that You Are a Spiritual Being

It is often the hectic pace of the world around us that makes us forget that we are spiritual beings living in a physical body. The world around us puts all the focus on our physical side and we end up forgetting the spiritual side.

To be well, you need a perfect balance between the two. If this balance is not in place, you feel incomplete, and fail to fulfill yourself.

Try to listen to both the needs of your body and your spirit, this will help you meditate better and maintain the balance in a stable way to feel good, complete, and fulfilled.

7. Focus on an Object

Training this practice in your daily life will be very helpful for you to focus better during meditation.

Choose an object that has meaning or significance to you and focus your attention on it for a few days. Using your senses explore it, but keep your attention on it only, and do it at least once a day. Focus on its color, its smell, and its texture to your touch. Does it have a taste? Does it reproduce a sound?

Use the power of focus and learn to concentrate. It will benefit you in your daily life and in meditation practice.

8. Perceive the Essence of the Object

After your focus and careful exploration of your chosen object, try to imagine its history.

Who produced it? Who touched it? Where did the materials that make it come from? Dig to find its true essence.

This search will send you deep into the nature of the object you are exploring and it will be a useful and important lesson for your meditation. During the practice, in fact, you have to go deeper and deeper inside yourself until you get in touch with your essence and with your true self. This object exercise will help you in your meditation practice.

9. Breathe

I have devoted a whole chapter to the relationship between breath and meditation, but I think in the tips for meditating better it is worth emphasizing its importance again.

Often, when you start meditating, you are plagued by various negative feelings. It may be that you start meditating to get rid of anxiety, fear, guilt, anger, sadness, or depression. These negative states, characterized by high tension, certainly do not make it easy for beginners to start. Breathing can really make a profound difference. Breathing correctly strongly helps to manage negative emotions. So, breathing slowly, calmly, and deeply will calm you down enough to get into the practice easier and to slip easier into the meditative state.

10. Don't be discouraged

If on your first attempts, you find it difficult to relax and clear your mind, and you keep getting distracted by a thought, it is because your mind is very active and thinks too much because of too many surrounding stimuli. I will elaborate on this concept in the next chapter, where I will be focusing on the most common mistakes.

It is important not to get discouraged and keep trying. With persistence and the various tips I share with you in this book, you will slowly begin to stay focused longer on the object of your meditation and you will notice when an extraneous thought is about to distract you, so you can let it flow without stopping it.

I repeat: Anyone can meditate!

11. Don't Give Yourself Deadlines

Don't give yourself deadlines by which you must have "learned" to meditate and time frames by which you expect to "see" the first results. These deadlines would end up generating a state of tension that would only complicate your approaches to meditation.

Learning to do anything well takes time and perseverance, and meditation is no exception. The problem is that the society we live in is primarily based on "everything right away" and on short-term results, so this may distort your perceptions.

Take as much time as you need and don't give yourself unnecessary deadlines.

The 13 Most Common Mistakes

In this chapter, I would like to address with you what I think are the biggest obstacles a beginner faces when deciding to start meditating. I am referring to those circumstances that make you say, "I don't know how to meditate," "It's not for me," or "I've tried, but I can't do it."

As I stated at the end of the introduction to this book: everyone can meditate and everyone should meditate. Everyone can do it; all it takes is the mind to meditate, and we all have one. Unfortunately, it is your mental schemes that hinder you in the process because they try to convince you that you are not capable. Your mental patterns keep telling you that you are making mistakes, that you are not doing it the right way, and that you should give up because you are not progressing at all. You listen to all this and you end up giving up. That's why I told you in the section on "Tips for getting started in meditation" that you should not judge yourself, so as not to trigger this mechanism.

Since I hear these negative statements too often, I decided to address the problem by defining the most common mistakes, to help you avoid falling into them or to get out of them promptly, should they happen to you. Let's see what prevents you from practicing correctly and why you are not getting all the benefits you can.

1. Your Mind is Too Restless

Just as it is true that during your day your mind is affected by the quality of your meditation, the opposite is also true. The amount of useless and stressful material you crowd your mind with every day and keep it occupied with, affects the quality of your meditation.

Meditation, I repeat, is a means to quiet your mind and keep its hectic activity in check. But, how can 5 minutes of meditation every now and then keep in check hours and hours of negative stimuli, mental stress, restlessness, and everything else you allow in into your mind for at least 12 hours a day every day? It would be like eating fast-food every day and expecting to weigh like a feather.

You should observe your mind during the day, try to understand what goes into it, and filter out some of the negative stimuli, for your own good. This will make it easier to meditate, and the better you meditate the calmer your mind will become, feeding a healthy circle that will bring you immediate benefits.

A mind that is too busy leads to the second problem.

2. Too Much Information

Most of what crowds your mind and makes it agitated and always busy comes from screens, which we have become accustomed to being glued to all day long. Social media, games, movies, news, blog articles, and I could go on much longer with this list.

In short, we expose our minds and brains to a flood of information for a very large number of hours every day, and when we sit down to meditate, our brains are in fervent activity. All this information gives us ideas, creates images and visions, and our brain and mental activity are overwhelmed with agitation.

Not only that, what is broadcasted on your screens is specifically designed to stimulate an emotional reaction in you, particularly related to 4 negative emotions: fear, anger, restlessness, and desire. Those 4 emotions agitate your mind as you try to learn how to meditate.

Again, how can a few minutes of sporadic attempts to learn how to meditate get the better out of hours of daily content that leverage such totalizing emotions?

You should analyze the emotions you feel when you consume certain content and, if you are stimulated by these negative emotions, you should reduce your viewing. This will improve your mental state and make it easier for you to deal with your first approaches to meditation, triggering the beneficial circle I mentioned earlier. You will meditate better, your mind will be calmer, and less hectic throughout the day, then you will meditate even better, and so on until you achieve inner peace and well-being in your life. You will be less stressed, more productive, and less distracted; you will be present in the "here and now."

These first two issues introduce the third.

3. You are Not Very Constant

Every day your mind is occupied with this huge amount of information and you often don't even find the constancy to meditate every day. It really only takes a few minutes a day to start getting results, but you don't find them, however, I bet you make time for your favorite social! It is time to choose and that is why I told you in the previous chapter that you need to find your why, you need a reason to be consistent.

To be permanently effective in your life, meditation must be practiced daily. If you sit and meditate once in a while you might enjoy some benefit on a physical level, but if you want real change in your life on a physical, mental, spiritual, and emotional level, you need daily constancy.

It really only takes even 2 or 3 minutes at first, but those 2 or 3 minutes have to be every single day because you have to develop a habit. This is how human beings function, we function by habits, we do what we do because we are used to doing it, and meditation has to become your habit.

Are your days too busy? Get up 5 minutes earlier! Not sure if you are doing it right? It doesn't matter, do it anyway, sooner or later you will get better. Not sure which technique you prefer? Pick one and get started. Nothing should stop your determination to meditate for 2 or 3 minutes daily.

You will see that slowly and without any effort on your part, those 2 or 3 minutes will become 5, then 10, and this too will start a positive circle of events. You will meditate better and without realizing it you will meditate longer, you will feel better, and meditate even better, and so on. So, your watchword is **CONSISTENCY**.

The fourth problem arises from a mix of the first three. Too much mental stimulation, too little constancy, and yet very high expectations.

4. You Have Unrealistic Expectations

It is right to start meditating because you are attracted by the benefits meditation brings to your life. It is wrong, however, to have unrealistic expectations and also to put all the focus on those expectations.

Until you seriously work on the first three mistakes mentioned you won't be able to see great results, so try not to fall into the mistake of giving up because you don't see the hoped-for benefits. It is just a matter of time, practice, and adjusting a few things along the way.

To solve this problem, it can help you not to put too much focus on expectations related to results. Try to focus on the pleasure that meditating gives you, and make the practice a fun, enjoyable time where you feel good.

5. You Don't Prepare Yourself

Many people struggle to enter a meditative state because they do not prepare to meditate. I have said many times that it only takes a few minutes a day to meditate, so don't expect a lot of preparation. It really only takes small gestures but they can make all the difference.

In step three of the steps on "How to start meditating", I indicated to you to take 3 deep breaths inhaling through the nose and exhaling through the mouth. This gesture is preparation because it relaxes and calms you, helps you to enter the meditative state more easily, and lets you go deeper with your meditation.

Some people prefer to state their intention instead of breathing, others need to stretch their muscles and loosen contractures, or practice various combinations of these three suggestions. You can experiment to find the best solution for you, the important thing is to prepare yourself in some way.

6. Too Much Confusion about Techniques

I devoted an entire chapter of this book to discussing the most popular meditation techniques and one chapter to recommending you a technique to start with.

Everyone is different, however, so once you have experimented with how to get started you should spend the first few weeks testing which technique is easiest for you to apply and which gives you the most results. Let's say that one week of testing each technique should be enough, and in just over a month you should have found your ideal solution.

Beginners often do not do this path of test and analysis. Therefore, they find themselves jumping from one technique to another with little benefit after months of attempts.

It is essential to find your technique and dedicate yourself to it for an appropriate amount of time. You can evaluate changes and variations when your experience begins to grow, but doing so at the beginning proves to be a mistake and a hindrance. You can't master any technique because you don't give yourself the time to do so and therefore you believe you are not capable of meditating.

Repetition of a technique, whether it is focusing on a chakra, mantra, or breath, makes you gain more intimacy and affinity with the technique itself. It will become easier and easier for you to practice it, your meditation will become deeper and deeper, and you will get better and better results.

So, give yourself a few weeks to choose the technique and then focus only on the chosen one.

7. You Doubt Too Much

As I mentioned in mistake 6, when you go from one technique to another and see no results, you start to persuade yourself that you are not capable of meditating. This doubt and self-criticism, in addition to demotivating you, tend to distract you during your practice.

Try not to judge yourself, especially during practice. As you practice, let yourself go, immerse yourself in meditation, and don't think about whether you are doing it right or wrong. Just do it.

All you have to do is focus your attention on the breath, a mantra, or a chakra and hold this attention as long as possible. When it fails, as soon as you notice it, bring it back to where you want it to be. At first, your attention will be short-lived and it will take you a while to notice that it is wandering, but with practice, you will hold it longer and longer and notice a lot quicker when it begins to wander.

No judgments, no doubts, just keep repeating this process, and your results will come. It may sound simplistic, but the gist of meditation is all here, in the brief process of keeping your attention as long as possible on the chosen object, and bringing it back as soon as you notice that something has distracted your concentration.

8. You Punish Yourself

A consequential mistake of doubting and judging yourself is that you punish yourself in some way. When a thought comes to distract you during meditation, you berate yourself.

Don't! It doesn't help your meditation and it doesn't help you. When a thought comes to distract you, welcome it, let it flow, and watch it go away without reproaching yourself for anything. Then, return your attention to the object of your meditation.

9. You Do not Practice with Attention

If you practice superficially and without paying due attention to your gestures, it is normal to find it hard to get into a meditative state, and you will hardly see any results. While practicing, you need to set aside thoughts such as the things you will have to do during the day. You have to concentrate only on meditation in that handful of minutes devoted to it; you have the rest of the day for other thoughts.

I think it's easy for you to understand this point because it applies a little bit to anything you do. If you do something carelessly and listlessly, you cannot expect results in any area.

10. You Don't Practice with Intention

You must practice meditation not only with attention but also with the intention to make it deeper and deeper. If you lack this element, you will find it difficult to find the necessary calm and commit yourself to the practice daily.

Try not to experience meditation as one of the many tasks of the day. Practice it with the intention of making an important gesture for you, the most important gesture of your day. It is an appointment with yourself and your well-being. Living it with this intentionality and with this kind of reverence will help you become better and better at it.

11. You Have no Patience

Certainly, meditation will help you develop this virtue, but you have to be patient if you want to learn to meditate.

You have to be patient with yourself and with the practice. You can and will get incredible results, but it will take time.

12. You Confuse Meditation and Relaxation

To meditate you have to relax, but, as I explained in the chapter on what meditation is, you have to "achieve a state of peace while still remaining alert." This means that meditating and relaxing are not synonymous.

To meditate properly you have to create a state of balance between relaxing and being alert. Do not confuse the two terms, otherwise by using relaxation as the only parameter, you might think you are not meditating, when in fact you are.

13. You Have Negative Thoughts

Many people think they are not meditating because some negative thought happens to cross their mind. Meditation helps you deal with negativity, and over time you will see the results. However, especially in the beginning, it is normal for some negative thoughts to cross your mind.

Don't worry about it and don't dwell on it. Just let it flow as you do with all other thoughts and stay focused on the object of your meditation. If you find that you dwell on it, don't reproach yourself, don't judge yourself, move on, let it go, and bring your attention back to the object of your meditation.

Step-By-Step Meditations

At this point in the book, you have enough information to successfully take your first steps into the world of meditation, and also a good amount of suggestions for moving to a more advanced level.

In this chapter, I would like to address meditation suggestions based on the time you have available or the purpose for which you are meditating. I will divide each practice into numbered steps and give you the outline of various guided meditations to make your approaches to the practice even easier.

On my YouTube channel, whose link is in the introduction, I often post guided meditations that you can follow, but having this written option has two additional functions. As I mentioned to you earlier, guided meditations are useful for beginners, especially those who are just starting out. However, this is not a truth that applies to everyone. For some, meditation is a very intimate process and, especially in the beginning, you want to do it in absolute solitude. For me, for example, this was the case. My first few times were in absolute solitude and autonomy, with time and experience, I was able to open myself to the teachings of a master and his guided meditations.

The second strength of these transcriptions is that they allow you to maintain intimacy while still giving you the precise directions you need, and you can leverage this information in two ways.

You can memorize the various passages and then perform them later. Or, with the voice recorder on your cell phone, you can record yourself slowly reading the various steps and build your own guided meditation, with your own voice and your own meditation times. As your only caution, I recommend that you allow time between steps to apply what you describe. In this way, you will also create a meditation of a length equivalent to the time you set for your practice, whereas in classic guided ones, the time is not set by you and, especially in the beginning, they can be a bit too long and tiring.

Well, if you are ready, let's begin.

Short Meditation - 1 Minute

Let's start with a very short meditation. It is simple and you can easily practice it every day. It only takes 1 minute to practice it and you do it by creating a connection with yourself and your breath. With regular practice, you will soon see the first benefits in your life.

You can also practice it for more than 1 minute, of course. However, even one minute repeated every single day will give you a deep sense of calm and balance and help you center and ground yourself.

Here are the steps to follow:

1. Sit on the floor, with your legs crossed and your back straight (with all your Chakras aligned), but relaxed. (If you prefer to sit on a chair or use a cushion that's okay too, just follow the directions in the chapter on "How to start meditating"). You need to be comfortable, but not too comfortable because you need to remain alert.

2. Shoulders relaxed, chest open, and hands laying on your thighs or knees.

3. Close your eyes. Breathe through your nose.

4. Focus on your breathing.

5. Start breathing in a controlled way and count the duration of your breath. Breathe in one, slow, deep stream, and make inhalation and exhalation the same time length. I recommend 3 or 4 seconds (for me 4

seconds is perfect). So, for example, inhale for 4 seconds and exhale for 4 seconds, then again. Inhale for 4 seconds and then exhale for 4 seconds. Continue ...

6. Focus all your attention on this count and let the breathing absorb you completely. Continue for one minute or as long as you decided to devote yourself to meditation. You are now breathing in a well-balanced way. As you follow the flow of your breath, feel the air entering your nose and reaching your whole body, and then leaving it as you exhale. Following your breath brings you into the present moment, into the "here and now", and infuses your body and spirit with calm and peace, making you feel grounded and balanced. Following your breath brings you into the present moment, centers, and roots you, and as you proceed with the practice, you feel it more and more deeply. Feel the balance between your body and mind.

7. Start by slowly moving the fingers of your hands to gradually move out of the state and go back to your body. Then slowly open your eyes. Before getting up, take a second to enjoy the feelings of peace, tranquility, and balance that you have generated, so that they will follow you as long as possible throughout your day, making it a better day.

The incredible advantage of this short meditation is that you can practice it virtually anywhere. In the office, sitting at your desk. On the subway, sitting on your way to work. At home, returning from a hard day. During a break, during an anxious moment, or during a particularly nerve-wracking or stressful circumstance. Allowing yourself to be completely absorbed by the breath as this meditation teaches you to do will calm you down, and give you the balance you need to deeply enjoy your day.

Short Meditation - 3 Minutes

This is another practice that aims to bring peace, serenity, and balance to your body and mind quickly. It only takes 3 minutes a day, every day, but, again, you can practice for as long as you want.

Here are the steps to follow:

1. Sit on the floor with your legs crossed and your back straight (with all your Chakras aligned), but not stiff. Relax your shoulders. (If you prefer to sit on a chair or use a cushion that's okay too, just follow the directions in the chapter on "How to start meditating"). You need to be comfortable, but not too comfortable because you need to remain alert.

2. Close your eyes. Breathe through your nose.

3. Shoulders relaxed, chest open, and hands laying on your thighs or knees.

4. Do not control your breathing. Breathe normally, and let your breath flow naturally.

5. Watch your breath flow because it brings you into the present moment, into the "here and now." Through the breath, relax your body, and let go of all tension. Do not hold any tension, let it go with your breath.

6. Keep observing your breath going in and out of your body. Visualize the exact process of the air entering your nose and traveling throughout your body when you inhale, and then leaving when you exhale. Continue for 3 minutes to stay focused on this observation and visualization of the air going in and out of your body.

7. If during this observation of your breath you get distracted or any thoughts come into your mind, that's okay. As soon as you notice it, bring your attention back to your breath and to your visualization of the air coming in through your nose, going through your whole body, and then leaving your body through your nostrils.

8. Start slowly moving your fingers on your hands to gradually come out of the state and return to your body.

Then slowly open your eyes. Before getting up, take a second to enjoy the feelings of peace, tranquility, and balance that you have generated, so that they will follow you as long as possible throughout your day, making it a better day.

Short Meditation - 5 Minutes

This practice too aims to bring peace, serenity, and balance to body and mind, pretty quickly. It only takes 5 minutes a day, every day, but, again, you can practice for as long as you want.

Here are the steps to follow:

1. Sit on the floor with your legs crossed and your back straight (with all your Chakras aligned), but not stiff. Relax your shoulders. (If you prefer to sit on a chair or use a cushion that's okay too, just follow the directions in the chapter on "How to start meditating"). You need to be comfortable, but not too comfortable because you need to remain.

2. Close your eyes. Breathe through your nose.

3. Shoulders relaxed, chest open, and hands laying on your thighs or knees.

4. Do not control your breathing. Breathe normally, and let your breath flow naturally.

5. Watch your breath flow because it brings you into the present moment, into the "here and now", and brings you awareness.

6. As you observe your breath flow, you can feel the air around you protecting you, wrapping around you, and supporting you.

7. As you watch your breath flow, you can feel the connection with Mother Earth supporting and protecting you. You can feel Her under you if you are sitting on the ground or under your feet if you are in a chair.

8. As you watch your breath flow, feel protected and supported by the Air and the Earth. Stay focused and concentrated on these sensations throughout your practice.

9. Begin by slowly moving the fingers of your hands to gradually move out of the state and back to your body. Then slowly open your eyes. Before getting up, take a second to enjoy the feelings of peace, tranquility, and balance that you have generated, so that they will follow

you as long as possible throughout your day and make it a better day.

All three of these practices can be practiced for different lengths of time. The real difference lies in which of the three makes you feel more comfortable and allows you to enter a meditative state more easily: breath control, observing your breath, or focusing on sensations. Testing the various methods will help you get to know yourself better and clearly understand what works for you.

Short Meditation for Gratitude - 5 Minutes

It only takes 5 minutes a day, every day, but, again, you can practice it for as long as you want. It is very similar to the other meditations already described, with the difference that you give yourself an intention, we might say a purpose. For example, your intention might be to be present, to be the observer of your breath, to be the observer of your energy, the observer of your body sensations, and so on. This practice brings calm, inner peace, and deep gratitude.

Here are the steps to follow:

1. Sit on the floor with your legs crossed and your back straight (with all your Chakras aligned), but not stiff. Relax your shoulders. (If you prefer to sit on a chair or use a cushion that's okay too, just follow the directions in

the chapter on "How to start meditating"). You need to be comfortable, but not too comfortable because you need to remain alert.

2. Close your eyes. Breathe through your nose.

3. Shoulders relaxed, face relaxed, chest open, and hands laying on thighs or knees.

4. Do not control your breathing. Breathe normally and let the breath flow naturally.

5. Watch your breath flow because it brings you into the present moment, into the "here and now", and makes you feel centered and grounded.

6. Bring your hands together in front of your chest and state your intention for this meditation. It could be, for example, to be present in the "here and now," present to yourself and your spirit. Choose your intention.

7. Become an observer of the present moment without judging yourself and state your intention, around or on your mind (whichever makes you more comfortable). Now you can put your hands back on your thighs or knees.

8. Go back to observing your breath, observing each time the air goes in and out of your body. Leave it natural and relaxed, just observe it. If you get distracted or a thought comes to your mind, bring your attention back to observing your breath as soon as you notice your distraction. Do this with intention, without judging, or punishing yourself.

9. Continue to observe your breath, bring your attention back to it throughout the practice, and allow the practice to make you feel peaceful and calm.

10. Before concluding the practice, bring your joined hands back to your heart level and express gratitude for all the reasons for gratitude that certainly abound in your life and that you can surely see more clearly in this state. Then carry all this gratitude with you after the practice and throughout your day.

11. Take a deep breath. Smile. Begin to slowly move your fingers to gradually come out of the state and return to your body. Then slowly open your eyes. Before getting up, take a second to enjoy the feelings of peace, calm, and gratitude that you have generated, so that they will follow you as long as possible throughout your day, making it a better day.

Short Morning Meditation - 3 Minutes

To start your day in the best way possible.

Here are the steps to follow:

1. Sit on the floor with your legs crossed and your back straight (with all your Chakras aligned), but not stiff. Relax your shoulders. (If you prefer to sit on a chair or use a cushion that's okay too, just follow the directions in the chapter on "how to start meditating"). You need to be comfortable, but not too comfortable because you need to remain alert.

2. Close your eyes. Breathe through your nose.

3. Shoulders relaxed, face relaxed, chest open, and hands laying on thighs or knees.

4. Do not control your breathing. Breathe normally and let your breath flow naturally.

5. Watch your breath flow through your body. Observe the air entering and leaving your body. Observe how cool the one entering your nose is and how warm the one coming out is. Observe the whole journey that oxygen makes through your body and takes root in it. Bring all your

attention inward, to the breath. This will root you in the present moment, into the "here and now".

6. Now observe the sensations generated in your body. Analyze each part of your body and how it feels to be in contact with the Earth underneath you, or the air around you. What sensations do those parts feel? They should all be pleasant sensations. If you feel a tightening somewhere, you need to control your breath and send your breath where you feel that knot. Your breath can loosen the knot and create a relaxed space in its place.

7. Feel present in your body, in your spirit, and into the world. Find yourself. Be present and aware. Practice this meditation for at least 3 minutes or as long as you like.

8. Take a deep breath. Smile. Start slowly moving your fingers on your hands to gradually come out of the state and return to your body. Then slowly open your eyes. Before getting up, take a second to enjoy the relaxing sensations you have generated, keep smiling, and let the smile and the relaxation follow you to get your day off to the best possible start.

Meditation for Better Sleep - Short - 5 Minutes

This short meditation prepares you for sleep and helps you enjoy deep sleep because it empties the mind and relaxes the body. It should be practiced just before going to sleep. It is very useful for those who struggle to get to sleep, those who have little restful sleep, those who cannot leave behind the weight of the day, and those whose minds are very active even when it is time to go to bed. It only takes 5 minutes of daily practice to improve the quality of your sleep but you can practice it even longer, depending on your needs. I recommend not practicing it by already lying down in bed. You should always practice it in a sitting position so that your chakras are aligned and your energy can flow freely.

Here are the steps to follow:

1. Sit on the floor with your legs crossed and your back straight (with all your Chakras aligned), but not stiff. Relax your shoulders. (If you prefer to sit on a chair or use a pillow that's okay too, just follow the directions in the chapter on "How to start meditating"). You need to be comfortable.

2. Close your eyes. Breathe through your nose.

3. Shoulders relaxed, face relaxed, chest open, and hands laying on your thighs or knees.

4. Do not control your breathing. Breathe normally and let your breath flow naturally.

5. Feel your body relax with your breath. Each time you exhale feel your body relax and your shoulders lower toward the ground.

6. Then, each time you exhale, bring softness into your body. Feel your joints become softer, all the tissues of your body, and then all your muscles from top to bottom. Feel your face soften when you exhale, feel your shoulders soften when you exhale, and also the heart area. Continuing down, feel your abdomen soften when you exhale, then your legs, and your feet.

7. Keep breathing flowing naturally, feel this sensation of softness throughout your body, and every time you exhale let go of any residual tension and throw all your tensions out of your body. Let go of the events of the day, especially the ones you didn't enjoy. Let go of the list of things you couldn't complete that are waiting for you tomorrow. Stop thinking about the things you didn't do as you would have liked, let them go too.

8. When you have let go of everything, welcome gratitude for all that your body has allowed you to do, and experience this deep sense of gratitude. Connect to this gratitude, feel love toward it, and toward yourself. Be grateful and in love with yourself, your mind, your body, and your soul. Continue to feel this deep gratitude until the end of the practice by going deeper and deeper into yourself as your breathing continues to flow naturally. Every time you exhale you throw out all the tensions and everything you no longer need.

9. When you feel ready, slowly open your eyes, rise slowly, and try to maintain the state you are in. Go immediately to bed. As you walk towards it keep feeling gratitude, love, and peace. When you are in bed, go back to visualizing your breath, visualize yourself throwing out everything you don't need or want, and continue until you fall asleep.

Meditation to Reduce Anxiety - Short - 5 Minutes

The purpose of this meditation is to abandon fear and feel safe. Fear and feeling unsafe are the two main conditions that trigger anxiety. In this meditation, you will let go of those two negative feelings and regain mental calm. You only need a consistent practice of 5 minutes a day to improve your anxious state and the level of stress in your life. You will also find it very useful to practice it before a situation that usually makes you anxious, for example, an interview with the boss, a date with a new potential partner, a sport or social event where you need to perform at your best, or even an exam.

Here are the steps to follow:

1. Sit on the floor with your legs crossed and your back straight (with all your Chakras aligned), but not stiff. Relax your shoulders. (If you prefer to sit on a chair or use a cushion that's okay too, just follow the directions in the chapter on "How to start meditating"). You need to be comfortable, but not too comfortable because you need to remain alert.

2. Close your eyes. Breathe through your nose.

3. Shoulders relaxed, face relaxed, chest open, and hands laying on thighs or knees.

4. Do not control your breathing. Breathe normally and let your breath flow naturally.

5. Watch your breath flow because it brings you into the present moment, into the "here and now", and makes you feel centered and grounded. Focus on your breath and

feel the muscles in your body relax with your breath. Breathe in and, when you exhale, throw out all the tension. Become soft and begin to distinctly sense the floor beneath you and the air brushing against your skin, and surrounding your body.

6. Now that you perceive the boundaries of your body, begin to visualize a blue light coming closer and closer to you until it embraces you completely. Now, the boundaries of your body are completely wrapped in this blue light. The blue light is a safe place, a place where you are not afraid. Stay here, wrapped in the safe blue light for as long as you need. If a thought comes to distract you, let it go, and come back here, to your safe place. Stay focused on the blue light that surrounds you and feel the peace, calm, and safety it gives you for as long as you feel you need it.

7. Begin to slowly move the fingers of your hands to gradually come out of the state and then return to your body. Then slowly open your eyes. Before getting up, take a second to enjoy the feelings of peace, calm, and security that you have generated, so that they will follow you as long as possible throughout your day, making it a better day.

Meditation to Reduce Stress - 10 Minutes

The deep connection that this meditation creates causes you to feel centered, and grounded, and calms your mind. In such a state, you start to feel free from the grip of stress and will easily manage violent emotions such as anger or nervousness. Those bad emotions are often characterized by rigid body posture and negative thoughts crowding your mind like you couldn't push them away. The relaxation of body and mind that are given by this meditation allows you to better manage these negative aspects, push away negative thoughts easily, and bring positive benefits into your life throughout your day. With daily repetition, you will reduce stress in your life and live a happier life. This technique is very useful for learning to let go of everything you need to let go of.

Here are the steps to follow:

1. Sit on the floor with your legs crossed and your back straight (with all your Chakras aligned), but not stiff. Relax your shoulders. (If you prefer to sit on a chair or use a cushion that's okay too, just follow the directions in the chapter on "How to start meditating"). You need to be comfortable, but not too comfortable because you need to remain alert.

2. Close your eyes. Breathe through your nose.

3. Shoulders relaxed, face relaxed, chest open, and hands laying on your thighs or knees.

4. Start focusing on yourself the moment you close your eyes. Let go of other thoughts. Let go of distractions.

5. Concentrate and focus on your breath so that the mind starts to calm down. Follow your breath and focus on yourself until you feel connected to your deepest inner part.

6. Bring all your attention to your body. Observe your back. It is straight, with the Chakras aligned, but not rigid. Your face, shoulders, and arms are relaxed. Observe your chest as it opens and expands with each inhalation.

7. Bring your attention back to your breath and observe its flow. Do not try to control it, let it flow spontaneously, and naturally. Observe the air entering your nose when you inhale and leaving when you exhale. Exhale gently. Visualize your breath making its journey through your body.

8. Each time you exhale, let go of all that is negative, all that no longer serves you, and all that you need to let go of. Keep your attention on observing your breath throughout your meditation and feel yourself letting go each time you

exhale. If a thought or something else comes to distract your attention, don't worry, and don't judge yourself. Just let go of the distraction, watch it as it passes, as it proceeds to go past, and bring your attention back to the breath observation.

9. While you observe your breath, you will begin to feel present and connected in the "here and now" because you will begin to sense the boundaries of your body, the earth where it rests, and the air that surrounds and embraces it.

10. Start by slowly moving the fingers of your hands to gradually move out of the state and then back to the body. Then slowly open your eyes. Before getting up, take a second to enjoy the sensations you have generated. Try to feel what has changed in you after this meditation. Take in all the sensations and emotions that come in both body and mind and bring them with you throughout your day.

TIP: This meditation is very useful for stimulating the Third Eye Chakra. To do this, you will only need to slightly modify the phase of coming out of this meditative state. At step 10, after starting to move your fingers, rub your hands together until your palms are warm. Then bring your hands together, joined as if in prayer, and raise them to forehead height. Place your thumbs in the space between the eyebrows and begin massaging the area with small concentric movements. Continue for a minute or two, then slowly open your eyes and proceed with the rest of the directions in step ten. This gesture will lengthen your meditation by a few minutes but will bring additional benefits to your life and well-being.

Mind-Body Connection Meditation - 5 Minutes

This practice helps you to connect your body and mind. It gives you a strong awareness of yourself, your body, your spiritual energy, and your immense and infinite potential. It is very useful for those who have problems with insecurity, fragility, and vulnerability because it helps the connection with the true and perfect self and its infinite energy. It is also very useful for balancing and energizing your Chakras, as the visualization you practice runs through your body's energy centers activating and stimulating them.

Here are the steps to follow:

1. Sit on the floor with your legs crossed and your back straight (with all your Chakras aligned), but not stiff. Relax your shoulders. (If you prefer to sit on a chair or use a cushion that's okay too, just follow the directions in the chapter on "How to start meditating"). You need to

be comfortable, but not too comfortable because you need to remain alert.

2. Close your eyes. Breathe through your nose.

3. Shoulders relaxed, face relaxed, chest open, and hands laying on thighs or knees. Arms are also relaxed so don't keep them stiff.

4. Bring attention to your breath and observe its flow. Don't try to control it, let it flow spontaneously, and naturally. Observe the air entering your nose when you inhale and leaving when you exhale. Breathe in a gentle, light, calm, and relaxed way. Visualize the breath making its journey through your body.

5. As you continue to observe the breath, begin to look inside yourself. Bring all your attention to the space in the center of your head. Slowly descend through your body keeping your attention on this journey. Bring your attention to your throat, then your chest, your heart, continue down to reach your navel, then your pelvis, and finally the part in contact with the ground. Keep constant awareness of this path, and when you have reached your bottom, slowly begin to walk back this same path the other way around, from your bottom to the top of your head.

6. When you have returned to the center of your head become aware that you are in a special place, through which you express your true being and your uniqueness. Gain a deeper and deeper awareness of your body and perceive it as it expands into the surrounding reality. Feel your immense greatness and your energy spreading everywhere.

7. Now your physical body is totally relaxed and deeply connected to your internal energy, and to your mind.

8. Begin to slowly move the fingers of your hands to gradually come out of the state and return to your body. Then slowly open your eyes. Before getting up, take a second to enjoy the sensations you have generated so that they will follow you as long as possible throughout your day, making it a better day.

Meditation to Calm Your Mind - 10 Minutes

Calming your mind is essential for maintaining well-being in times of stress, anxiety, or when you are affected by a negative or emotionally frustrating event. This practice is therefore very useful in a varied number of circumstances, for example, for those who work in a difficult and competitive environment, for those who are experiencing a difficult relationship, for those who are having difficulties in their relationships with their family, and in general, in all those situations that generate negative feelings that cause anxiety, stress, outbursts of anger, or feelings of unmotivated sadness. The practice involves the recitation of the "Sacred Mantra of Breath". The empty space between the recitation of the two verses of the mantra creates a deep sense of peace, which is why this technique succeeds in calming the mind so effectively.

Here are the steps to follow:

1. Sit on the floor with your legs crossed and your back straight (with all your Chakras aligned), but not stiff. Relax your shoulders. (If you prefer to sit on a chair or use a cushion that's okay too, just follow the directions in the chapter on "How to start meditating"). You need to be comfortable, but not too comfortable because you need to remain alert.

2. Close your eyes. Breathe through your nose.

3. Shoulders relaxed, face relaxed, chest open, and hands laying on thighs or knees. Arms are also relaxed so don't keep them stiff.

4. Relax your whole body, trying to ground, and center yourself in this relaxed position.

5. Bring your attention to your breath and observe its flow. Don't try to control it, let it flow spontaneously, and naturally. Observe the air entering your nose when you inhale and leaving when you exhale. Breathe in a gentle, light, calm, and relaxed way. Visualize the breath making its journey through your body.

6. As your breath flows freely, begin to visualize a beach at the sea or lake. Observe the water and its fluidity. Be inspired by this element, by its fluidity, by the way, it always adapts to circumstances, and also by its strength and energy. Visualize the water enveloping you. This element is outside and inside you.

7. Keep observing your breath and associate a mantra with it. The sacred mantra of breath is "I AM". When you inhale, mentally pronounce "I", and when you exhale, mentally pronounce "AM". Mentally repeat the mantra with each breath. (TIP: For the beneficial effects of the mantra to occur you must keep a constant focus on your breath and bring back your attention immediately in case of any distraction. In addition, you can also use the original Sanskrit version of the mantra, which is "SO HAM", meaning precisely "I AM THIS". You will mentally repeat "SO" when you inhale and "HAM" when you exhale).

8. The mantra enters the body, goes through it, and flows through it. It is like a wave of water flowing through you with all its energy. Proceed with mental repetition of the mantra throughout the practice. Keep hearing it and visualizing it as a wave flowing through you, while keeping your attention on your breath. The sound of the mantra repeated in your mind sounds like a whisper produced by a little wave. This sound brings you to the present moment and you become the mantra.

9. Before leaving the state, let go of the mantra slowly and stay in your breath for a few seconds (count at least three deep breaths).

10. Start moving the fingers of your hands slowly to gradually exit the meditation state and return to your body. Then open your eyes slowly. Before getting up, take a second to enjoy the feelings you have generated so that they will follow you as long as possible throughout your day, making it a better day. Feel gratitude for yourself because you have taken time to devote to yourself, your well-being, and inner peace, bringing enormous benefit to your life.

TIP: You may find it pleasing to put audio in the background that reproduces the sound of waves of a calm sea.

Conclusion

Here we are at the end of this journey together!

I would really like to thank you for following me this far, and I hope it has been as enjoyable for you to go through this journey together as it has been for me to lead you to the discovery of the wonderful world of meditation and your inner power.

You now possess all the knowledge to begin practicing meditation successfully and unlock your inner power. I hope you have already started to test and look for the practice that suits you better.

Do not treat this book as pure entertainment or a means to satisfy a curiosity, please use it as the tool it is intended to be. I have written it to enable you to bring all the incredible benefits of meditation into your life in an easy way, and I really hope you will.

I would love to hear what you think of this book and if it has helped you in any way. A review would certainly be appreciated, but you can also contact me directly by email: comesbloccareituoichakra@gmail.com

You can also reach me on my YouTube channel, where you can write me in the comments of any video:

https://www.youtube.com/channel/UC5DxslTyhtdH5iQo1UtkO9Q

My channels are mainly in Italian because I am Italian and I started my teachings in my own country. Anyhow, feel free to write me in English. In fact, I am in touch with loads of English-speaking people that bought my books who seek advice now and again or enquire about new books coming out.

Finally, if you are interested in learning more about my content I leave you the link to my previous book, which I have often mentioned in various chapters. The title is, "Chakras for Beginners - A Complete Guide to Balance Your Chakras and Healing Yourself with Yoga, Meditation, Crystals, Essential Oils, and Other Self-Healing Techniques". Most of the topics are closely related to the ones I explained in this book. All my content is focused on taking care of yourself to improve the quality of your life emotionally, mentally, spiritually, and physically.

Ebook:

https://www.amazon.com/dp/B0B5PB7DB9

Paperback (color):

https://www.barnesandnoble.com/w/chakras-for-beginners-mind-body-masterclass/1141405006?ean=9781739665210

Hardcover (color):

https://www.amazon.com/dp/B0B5KV646F

Well, now it is really the time of farewells. I hope to see you again somewhere, be it an email, another book, or a video.

I wish you all the best in life,

NAMASTÉ

Anja D.

Book 2:

Chakras For Beginners

A Complete Guide to Balance Your Chakras and Healing Yourself with Yoga, Meditation, Crystals, Essential Oils, and Other Self-Healing Techniques

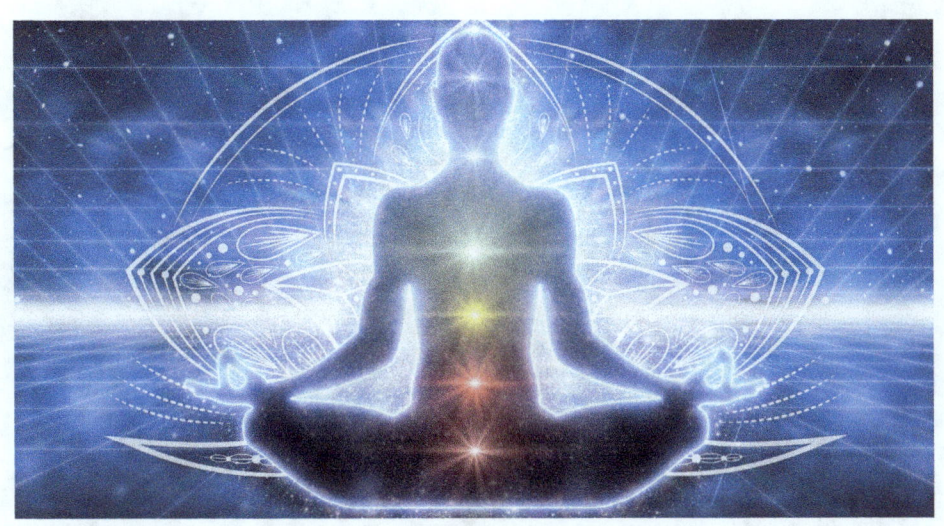

Introduction

It happens to all of us, in the course of life, to face difficult times, periods of deep frustration, and sad situations that mark us deeply. At these junctures, we yearn to find the serenity and tranquility lost. To do so, we start looking for desperate solutions or magic remedies.

We look for practical remedies, then we move on to spiritual ones, but often the discomfort we feel is so deep that we do not notice that we are taking information from the wrong sources or that we are relying on the advice of unreliable people, and this only makes the situation worse.

This feeling of difficulty and discomfort that we feel inside is given by our energy that expresses itself in all its different aspects. The emotionality that we feel, the confusing feelings, the need for peace and serenity that we feel and that we are not able to reach, they all depend on our energy in that given moment.

The study of Chakras, which is the study of our energy, is the solution to understanding this feeling of emotionality and discomfort, and also to understand how this condition, in turn, causes negative consequences to our mind and then to our body.

By undertaking the study of the chakras you will no longer need to seek help from unreliable sources or wrong people. You will be able to identify for yourself the origin of your discomfort and alleviate your suffering until you eliminate it with the simple practices related to this discipline.

To understand what the Chakras are and how they work, you will have to imagine your body as a big container full of many small spheres made of energy and connected by a constant flow of energy. All these spheres are your Chakras. Among all those spheres there are 7 that are larger and have more energy than all the others, and all this energy makes them glow more than all the others. These 7 spheres are vertically aligned with each other and are the 7 Main Chakras.

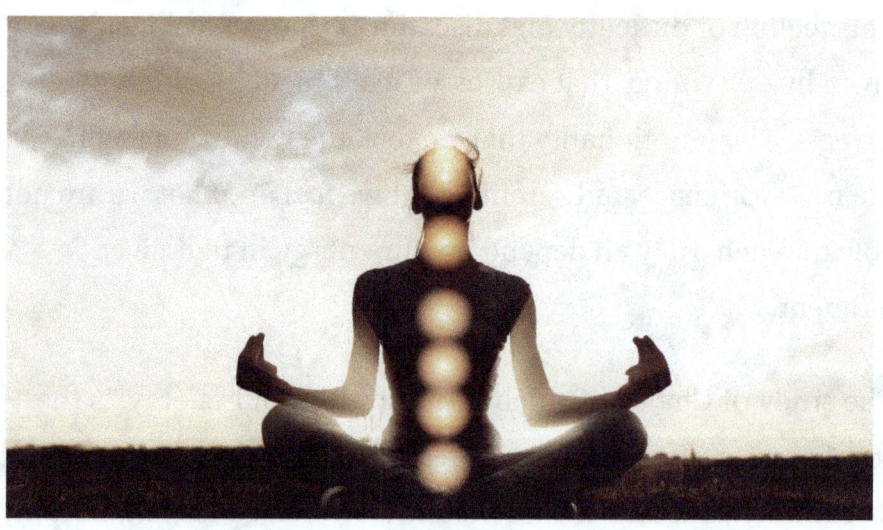

The energy flowing through these spheres emits invisible but easily perceivable vibrations. Depending on the energy flowing through these spheres, the vibrations can be positive or negative.

I said that these vibrations are invisible but easily perceived and I am sure you understand exactly what I am talking about. I'm sure it has happened to you hundreds of times to enter an environment such as a room, a party hall, or a restaurant and immediately feel anxiety or discomfort, rather than joy or happiness. The people present in that environment may have a big smile on their faces, but the energy doesn't lie, and if you have felt anxiety and discomfort, those are the vibrations that those people are spreading in the environment.

I mentioned earlier that these vibrations can be positive or negative based on the energy flowing. I'm not just referring to the quality of the energy, but also to the quantity of energy. If something blocks our energy and it cannot flow freely, we experience all the various problems discussed at the beginning of this introduction: frustration, sadness, discomfort, emotionality, ... along with all the mental and physical consequences related.

Therefore, learning about your Chakras, how to unlock their energy, and how to balance it will allow you to heal these discomforts. If you make these practices of unblocking, healing, and balancing the energy of the Chakras part of your daily life, you will enjoy very long periods of well-being and you will truly never again need to go looking for magical solutions from the wrong sources.

Immerse yourself in the study of Chakras, in the study of your own energy. It will allow you to take control of your life and direct it towards the happiness and peace that you deserve and want. You can improve relationships with people you care most for and those around you. More generally, you can improve your relationship with the world around you.

In order to keep the Chakras open and functioning, it is necessary to understand what may be causing the blocks that interrupt or reduce the flow of energy. In the in-depth analysis of each of the 7 main Chakras, we will go into detail about the specific causes of blockage of each specific Chakra, but I think it is very important to illustrate what I consider a fundamental element for understanding the problem.

The causes of energy that does not flow properly or is blocked can be many. For example, having bad habits or not taking proper care of your body can be the main cause of the malfunctioning of our energy centers. There are 2 elements in particular, however, that I believe to be the major causes of

Chakras blockage: continually trying to repress yourself to be different from what you are and negativity, negative energy expressed through negative emotions.

Trying to show to be different from what you really are so that you are closer to a socially acceptable ideal causes anxiety, depression, and mental and emotional stress. All these negative feelings lead us to the second cause of Chakras' blockage.

When I speak of negative feelings or emotions, however, I am not just referring to yours. Your energy centers pick up energy from the world around you, so they also pick up the negative vibrations of the people around you who are plagued by negative emotions. As you can see, it's not just a matter of knowing how to handle your negative emotions, but more importantly, choosing well the people you surround yourself with. Doing an excellent job on yourself and then hanging out with people who radiate negativity would negate all your good work. Not only that but by associating with these people you would end up passing through or staying in places impregnated with those negative vibrations that would further block your flow of positive energy.

In the next chapters, you will understand how to work well on your Chakras but accept the advice to choose carefully the people with whom you hang around and the places you frequent.

Don't be afraid of not knowing how to choose, as you read these lines you probably already have negative places or people in mind. You know this because when you meet them you feel a sadness that you can't explain, or you reach the house of "a friend" and feel an unfounded sense of unease. Trust your energetic sphere and clean your surroundings of toxic people and places and you will see the first benefits immediately.

How Do Chakras Work?

I mentioned in the introduction that Chakras are spheres of energy connected by a constant flow of energy. But where does this energy come from? Chakras allow the energy of the external world to enter and flow within us. I used the similarity with the spheres to introduce the Chakras because the translation of the Sanskrit term is "circle" or "wheel".

You can imagine Chakras as small luminous wheels in perpetual movement that receive energy from the external world and expand it in a constant flow within each one of us. This energy flowing within each one of us, allows our body to perform all its functions on the physical level, the mental level, the spiritual level, and the emotional level, that is, on all four "layers" of the human being.

These little wheels of energy in our body, our Chakras, are hundreds in number. It is essential for our wellness on all four levels of our being that the energy that enters our body flows abundantly and constantly through all those wheels. Not all Chakras are the same, there are major and minor ones, but they must all allow the energy to flow appropriately. At the moment in which even only one of them does not carry out its function correctly, we immediately begin to experience symptoms.

Within the major and minor Chakras, we can identify seven Chakras that are called "The 7 Main Chakras". As I mentioned in the introduction, they are vertically aligned and we can visualize them in a vertical line that follows the spine from the base to the top of the head. Each of these 7 Chakras is positioned at an exact point of the spine.

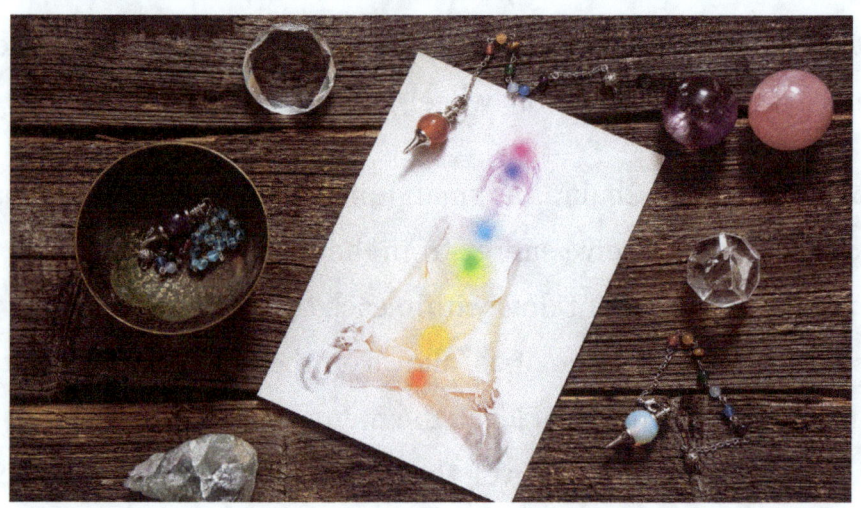

You will have understood by now that our whole daily life is influenced by our Chakras and their state of health. If our energy is not flowing as it should then our life will surely have problems.

In the following chapters, we are going to analyze in deeper detail the characteristics of each one of the 7 main Chakras, their causes of blockage, how to remove those blocks, and all the information you will need to bring harmony back into your life. The first step of this process, however, is awareness and you have already walked this first step by starting to study this manual. Being aware of the existence of the Chakras and knowing how to use them to your advantage, by keeping them open so that energy can flow freely, is the first step to maintaining good physical, mental, emotional, and spiritual health.

Chakras influence our daily life so deeply because they don't just take care of the energy in our physical body, but they act as a bridge connecting our body to the mind, the emotions, and the spirit. By the terms mind, emotions and spirit I am referring to the parts of the human body that are invisible to the senses. Each Chakra must work in harmony and balance with the others to create the ideal condition for our well-being. This ideal condition is a harmonic connection between our visible and invisible parts.

Each of the 7 main Chakras has, in fact, a physical correspondent such as an organ or a gland, and also a specific correspondence to certain aspects of our "invisible part". According to the Indian tradition, from which the Chakras originate, each of the 7 main Chakras is also linked to different colors, sounds, frequencies, mantras, images, and deities and it is because of these characteristics that each Chakra affects a different area of our daily life.

We spoke before about hundreds of spheres, while now we have reduced to 7 main Chakras. There are 2 other groups of Chakras, besides the 7 main ones.

In the second group, we find the so-called Minor Chakras, mainly located in the center of the palm of the hands, in the fingertips, in the linga, in some areas of our feet, and in some other areas.

The third group of Chakras includes all those of very small size or, even, tiny. They are so many to be practically incalculable, you can find one at each point where two energy lines meet.

We will deal with the opening, balancing, and unlocking of the 7 main ones. Basically, when the 7 Chakras work in harmony with each other, the ones belonging to the second and third groups just follow along.

The Origin of the Study of Chakras

The study of Chakras and their structure has very ancient origins. The original study of Chakras has its roots in India and the oldest evidence of this study are the Vedas, an ancient collection of popular sacred texts in Sanskrit. As for the historical period, we are between 1500 and 500 B.C. and originally the study of these "wheels" was handed down orally.

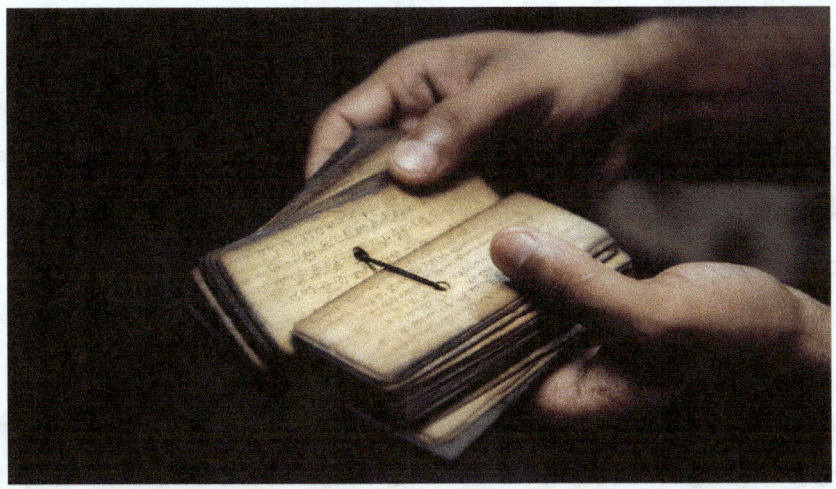

Western culture came across these ancient studies in 1919 with the book of Arthur Avalon, an English student of these disciplines, entitled "The Power of the Serpent". This book is considered the first document studying the application of

Kundalini Yoga. In the work, the author describes the philosophical and mythological nature of Kundalini and explains the anatomy associated with it, i.e. the energy centers of the human body (Chakras), their progressive awakening, and the Yoga poses and techniques associated with this practice of awakening. The most interesting part strictly related to the topic we are discussing, however, is that the book contains the translation of two ancient Indian documents that, until then, were considered secret and one of them is entirely dedicated to the study of Chakras.

From this important starting point, the study of Chakras has gone from being a subject for a few enthusiasts to a discipline of study for a wider audience. Most people now find this term quite familiar and feel comfortable with the study of this discipline and the benefits that its knowledge can bring to the life of each individual.

The 7 Main Chakras

Let's briefly recap what has been said so far. Chakras are spheres of energy in our body that are responsible for letting the energy in and making it flow from one point to another. They are located in a part of the body that is not perceptible to the senses. This part is called the "astral body" and is where the soul lives. The "astral body" is a part of the "subtle bodies", which are the layers of the human body that the senses cannot see or perceive. The "subtle bodies" are energy fields composed of etheric organs that have an equivalent on the physical plane with physical organs such as the heart, the liver, and so on.

The 7 main Chakras, therefore, are located in the "astral body" along the line of the spine, and, starting from the bottom and going upwards, they run along the whole spinal column. Each of them has an equivalent organ on the physical plane, therefore an organ of our body. Each Chakra transmits a specific vibration, associated with a certain color.

With this premise, it is easy to understand how the blockage of a Chakra can cause problems on a physical, mental, spiritual, and emotional level.

The functioning of the Chakras is quite simple. They take energy from the Universe, store it and then act as crossroads for its distribution. They make it flow towards all the adjacent Chakras in a constant and regular flow. As long as this condition of flow is respected, you will feel well physically, mentally, spiritually, and emotionally.

The moment one of these energy centers is blocked, a regular and constant flow of energy in your body will no longer occur, and as a result, various physical, mental, spiritual, or emotional problems will start to show up in your life. The type of problem will depend on which Chakra is not properly open, and therefore where the blockage and misalignment originates.

How can you tell if your Chakras are aligned or not? You simply need to analyze yourself to see if you have symptoms. We will go into more detail later, but I can start to give you some suggestions. Do you ever wake up with an unexplainable feeling of discomfort and unease? Do you often feel sad for no reason? Do you often feel strong, exaggerated, and uncontrolled feelings towards someone? Are you unable to express your creativity? Do you feel like you can never have fun? Do you have low self-esteem and constant fear of rejection? Do you suffer from hard-to-justify and uncontrollable outbursts of anger? Do you find it difficult to communicate with others whether it is in words or in writing?

I could go on with the list but these first questions should be enough to make you think about your actual situation. If you find yourself in one or more of the circumstances I have just described in my questions, then it is very likely that one of your Chakras is creating a blockage to your energy flow, and so your energy cannot proceed as it should, in a flux regular and constant.

It is fundamentally important to understand this process because with the awareness you gain you can decide to take action to remove the blockage. In the course of the book, you will understand how to identify which Chakra is responsible for what distress, and how to fix the problem. I would like to anticipate, however, that there are many methods to unlock and free your energy and you can choose the one you feel is more adaptable to you. Numerous Yoga positions allow the energy to flow, opening the Chakras and regulating their flow. Some massages perform a similar function. Furthermore, since each Chakra is associated with a color, gemstone, essential oil, and a certain vibration, you could choose to unblock your Chakras and rebalance them with color therapy, essential oils, and the use of particular minerals and gems. Meditation on its own, or accompanied by the repetition of Mantras or positive affirmations is also very useful.

Now let's go a little deeper into understanding each individual Chakra.

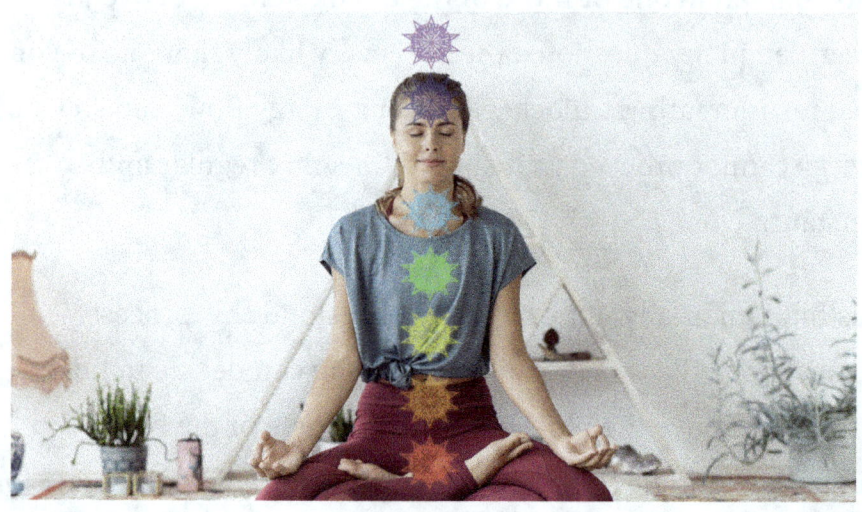

Each Chakra rotates at a different speed and has a different brightness according to the age of a person and his physical condition. So, brightness and rotation speed change using the course of a person's life because of the increasing ages, and because of the changing conditions, for example in case of stress or disease.

We have already said several times that when we look at the position of Chakras we move from the bottom to the top. We can identify the first three at the base of our spine moving up towards the head. They are the three lowest or "inferior" ones and are those related to the material needs and the fundamental needs of the human being. Included in this group of needs are food and nourishment, protection, economic security and, therefore, money, but also self-esteem, the need to be accepted, physical appearance, and sex.

The top three, moving up from the throat, are the "upper" and "higher" ones. They are more related to spirituality and otherworldly needs. This group of needs includes the search for the reason why we come into the world, the desire to evolve and improve, the desire to understand ourselves and others, but also ambition and the search for truth as opposed to illusion.

To regulate the lower and upper Chakras there is the Heart Chakra, the center of the entire energy system, the Chakra of love in all its forms, which aims to maintain a balance between soul, mind, and body.

Before moving on to the analysis of each Chakra I would like to emphasize once again that each Chakra corresponds to an organ of our body from the anatomical point of view. This means that, if the Chakra connected to a certain organ is blocked, the organ could not function correctly and could not perform its functions in a totally correct way. This malfunctioning could potentially lead your body into a state of disease and that is why it is essential to make sure that your Chakras are always open, and well balanced. In this way, your vital energy can flow properly leading you to enjoy physical, mental, spiritual, and emotional health.

The energy that flows in our body is called "Prana" in Indian philosophical terminology. This name comes from Sanskrit, a language in which the term "Prana" means life, but is also used with the meaning of "spirit" or "breath". Therefore, "Prana" is the vital energy that flows within and around us. Thanks to the "Prana", we communicate with the outside world in a constant exchange of energy and vitality, we take energy from the world around us and return it. This energy, "Prana", is connected to our Chakras, it's the energy that flows through your Chakras.

Now let's find out what the 7 main Chakras are, what they influence, which organs of the body they are identified with, what vibration and color they correspond to, and a lot more. You need this information because it is through these "rules" that the Chakras manage your life. Your energy flow is managed according to these basic criteria. You will be able to use this information to make a "diagnosis" about the state of each one of your Chakras.

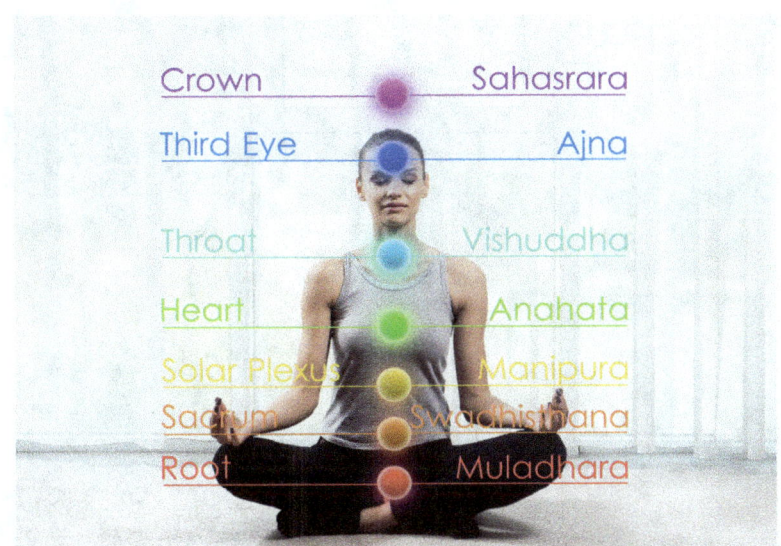

Root Chakra (1st)

(Sanskrit name: Mūlādhāra)

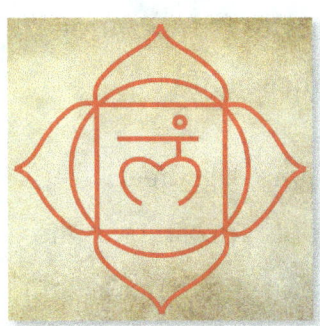

Element: Earth

Color: Red

Position: Coccyx

Planet: Mars

Characteristics of a well-balanced Chakra: It is called the Root Chakra because it is the root that connects us directly with the Earth, our mother. It keeps us constantly anchored to our material reality, makes us desire stability, and always have a contact and a connection with our roots. It is the Chakra of stability and is closely linked to the survival instinct and the basic needs of the human being. It is the Chakra of vitality and energy, regeneration of blood and tissues. It is responsible for giving a sense of security and stability, promoting destiny, and generating warmth. This Chakra also acts as a link with our past, our roots, and our ancestors. If it is well balanced we live our memories with harmony and without excessive attachment, we are not obsessed with the past, and we can live in the present, letting go of memories when necessary. The first Chakra gives us a strong instinct to survive and a balanced attachment to life, together with great respect for our body and our planet, necessary for our life and our survival.

Personal qualities related to this Chakra: Survival, being well-grounded, satisfaction, stability, instinctive trust, courage, vitality, power to achieve goals, full acceptance of life.

Which organs is it associated with? Spine, legs, feet, ankles, bones, coccyx, rectum, kidneys, bladder, prostate, male reproductive system, immune system, sense of smell, nose, skin, nails, teeth, and gums.

What physical problems is it related to? It is linked to physical problems that affect the intestine and the difficulty in the clearing, purifying, and eliminating toxins. There are frequent problems with the bones, legs, feet, and knees due to a bone structure that is not very solid. It is often associated with a stiff and not very fluid way of walking. It may cause problems with teeth, problems losing weight, problems with obesity, nervous anorexia, and even problems with the genital organs. Severe weakness for no reason is also common.

What part of the emotional sphere does it affect? Being this Chakra so deeply linked to human basic needs and instinct of survival, and self-preservation, it gives us the desire to live and experience the material world and what it has to offer. It makes us desire monetary autonomy, money through which we can meet the basic needs of feeding, clothing, and shelter. It makes us desire to put down roots in a place where we are happy, but it also makes us desire to change for a better and better life.

Symptoms of a blocked Chakra: First and foremost, you feel a sense of abasement and disconnection with your surroundings: you never feel at home anywhere. You feel chained to the surrounding environment, or to the people in your personal sphere because of low self-love and low self-esteem. A conflictual relationship with the mother figure is common. Usually, you never notice a specific reason as the cause of discomfort. Another symptom of the blockage of this Chakra is a strong sense of instability and difficulty in adapting to change. This internal and emotional discomfort manifests itself in some of the physical symptoms already described. Economic problems are also a clear symptom of the blockage of this Chakra, as well as doing a job that you do not like, and that does not give you stimulus or satisfaction.

Possible causes of blockage or imbalance: Too fearful or too greedy behaviors can be a primary cause. Pretending that everything is always fine, while inside we are oppressed by fear, can also be a cause of a blockage. Cultivating fear and continuing to blame ourselves for cultivating it are further obstacles to the flow of the Chakra's energy. Another cause of imbalance or blockage is the relationship between the person and his surrounding environment. In the definition of the surrounding environment, we can include all the people that revolve around the person himself, such as friends, family, partner, ... If the person is inserted in an environment that is wrong for him, here we have the problems described in the symptoms of the blocked Chakra. In this regard, if you feel judged by the people who make up your surrounding environment, this can lead to problems. In fact, if you hide your nature in order not to run into these judgments you create a strong obstacle to the flow of your energy.

Gems of the Root Chakra: The gems and stones that help to balance this Chakra are those of yellow-reddish color. The main one is red jasper, but it is also in tune with red agate and fire agate, red calcite, hematite, garnets, black onyx, fire opal, obsidian, ruby, smoky quartz, and brown zircon.

Associated colors: Red, brown, black, and gray

Associated sense: Olfaction

Associated fragrances: Cedar, sandalwood, cypress, patchouli, vetiver, and olibanum. These are strong, intense fragrance oils that are dark in color and have a woody or resinous scent.

Associated number: 4

Associated mantra: LAM

Associated foods: Foods that regulate body temperature, hot and energetic foods, such as chili peppers, tomatoes, radicchio, red onions, eggs, beets, meat, ... (mainly red foods).

Sacral Chakra (2nd)

(Sanskrit Name: Svadhishthana)

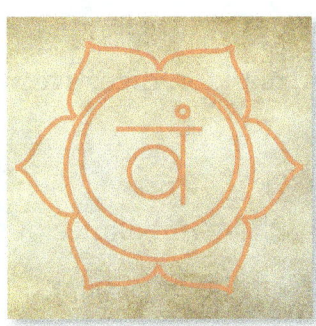

Element: Water

Color: Orange

Position: Below the navel (pubis)

Planet: Mercury

Characteristics of the well-balanced Chakra: Sexual creativity, balance, serenity, joviality, and spontaneity. The second Chakra influences our relationships with others, our sexuality, our pleasure and physical well-being, and the way we manage our emotions. Its foundation is pleasure and recognition for us from others. The second Chakra offers us a deep connection of harmony with nature that we see expressed in creative activities such as gardening, painting, photography, or even martial arts. To be in harmony with this Chakra means to be at peace with yourself, at ease and aware of your strengths and weaknesses, and to be magnetic and luminous people. It is the Chakra of our social instinct, of wanting to live among more people, and not alone.

Personal qualities related to this Chakra: Primary feelings, sexuality, desire, sensuality, pleasure, relationships, admiration, union with nature, openness, transparency, and personal creativity.

Which organs is it associated with? Ovaries, testicles, reproductive system, small intestine, spleen, bladder, digestive and intestinal system, and sciatic nerve.

What physical problems is it related to? The imbalance of this Chakra is linked to sexual or reproductive problems, back pain in the pelvic area, and disorders in the kidneys and urination.

What part of the emotional sphere does it affect? This Chakra influences the ability to express love, but also one's ability to express desires, creativity, and have fun along the way. When balanced we are pervaded by creativity, confidence, and passion. It is the Chakra that is the home to all of our emotions. These emotions can be positive or negative based on previous experiences and also based on the social context, family, and friends around us.

Symptoms of a blocked Chakra: The main symptom is a lack of confidence mainly in oneself and continuous unfounded fears. There are frequent emotional blocks, low passion, absence of libido, and creativity in all its forms. For example, we fail to connect with our passions, or we lack the enthusiasm to do so. In some cases, we feel a spasmodic need to keep all aspects of our lives under control, and we lack love and self-esteem. We fail to connect with others, even in intimacy. Weakness, exhaustion, and feeling lacking in gifts or talents are all very clear symptoms of energy blockage in this Chakra. Fear, anger, and anxiety dominate us when this Chakra is not functioning well, often resulting in a sense of depression. We experience life as a kind of struggle where we are alone to face everyone, and can never find serenity.

Possible causes of blockage or imbalance: Emotional trauma, constant stress, and too sedentary life are the main causes of blockage. Feelings of guilt are another cause of strong blockage of this Chakra's energy. The feeling of guilt is associated with the feeling of being imprisoned because you don't want to take responsibility for your life and, therefore, getting rid of want doesn't do you any good. On a physical level, the blockage of energy can be caused by abuse of our body, for example, if we stress it with continuous negative thoughts, or if we mistreat it with the consumption of alcohol, and cigarettes.

Gems of the Sacral Chakra: The main gem of this Chakra is the Carnelian, the stone of mental and spiritual pleasure. It is however in tune with most stones in shades of orange such as amber, moonstone, fire opal, and orange calcite.

Associated color: Orange

Associated sense: Taste

Associated scents: Jasmine, orange, gardenia, ylang-ylang, pine, birch, and juniper. These are less strong essential oils than those of the first Chakra, with a strong aphrodisiac power, or the power to stimulate purification.

Associated number: 6

Associated mantra: VAM

Associated foods: The foods of this Chakra are those naturally sweet, rich in minerals, and aphrodisiacs such as oranges, mandarins, pumpkin, saffron, carrots, and mangoes, apricots, honey, coconut, oats, sesame, cinnamon ... (mainly orange food).

Note: the passing of too much energy through this Chakra can cause excessive lust, addiction in various forms, and an excessive sense of control. This makes it critical that the flow of energy is constantly kept balanced.

Solar Plexus Chakra (3rd)

(Sanskrit name: Manipura)

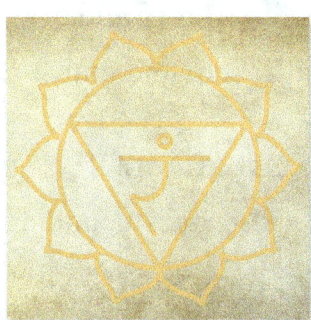

Element: Fire

Color: Yellow

Position: Above the navel

Planet: Jupiter

Characteristics of the well-balanced Chakra: This Chakra carries the power of wisdom and knowledge. It controls our ego. It makes us aware of our new physical and mental potential. It helps us to be who we really want to be. It promotes digestion and gives access to happiness and self-confidence. It allows us to assimilate energy. It gives us tranquility, respect, and dignity towards ourselves. Its main purpose is our self-acceptance. It is the Chakra responsible for our actions and our intentionality.

Personal qualities related to this Chakra: Personal power, strength, authority, self-control, peace, joy, inner harmony, self-acceptance, social identity.

Which organs is it associated with? Pancreas, nervous system, digestive system, liver, spleen, large intestine, stomach, transverse colon, gallbladder, metabolism, muscles, and eyes.

What physical problems is it related to? Disorders of the liver, stomach, pancreas, gallbladder, and colon. Ulcers and gastritis are frequent. Bloating. Problems with teeth and gums.

What part of the emotional sphere does it affect? It affects the emotional sphere of self-esteem, self-criticism, and our relationship with power.

Symptoms of a blocked Chakra: Strong selfishness, deep states of anxiety, sense of shame, and problems related to self-assertion on the physical, mental, and emotional levels. For example, it manifests in the form of a fear of rejection or criticism for one's physical appearance. This creates a tendency to isolate oneself and avoid contact with others. You feel inadequate, powerless, and unable to achieve your goals. Everything seems like an insurmountable obstacle. Anger is repressed rather than expressed, causing deep mental distress that spills over into the body causing illness.

Possible causes of blockage or imbalance: A poor care of our image could be the main cause of the imbalance of this Chakra. This is true on the outer level and it is expressed in the way we dress, in the way we take care of our bodies, and in the way we take care of our physical form. It is also true on the emotional and intellectual level and it is expressed by the fact that we don't have goals to achieve or that we don't celebrate our victories and successes. The tendency to suppress our abilities and talents can also be an obstacle to the flow of energy through this Chakra. Feelings of frustration and shame are major obstacles to its balanced energy flow. We never pause to analyze the causes of negative, deleterious, and destructive emotions, thus aggravating the blockage.

Gems of the Solar Plexus Chakra: The main stone is citrine quartz. This Chakra is however attuned to yellow stones such as gold, yellow zircon, pyrite, yellow opal, tiger's eye, imperial topaz, and sulfur.

Associated colors: Yellow and gold

Associated sense: Sight

Associated fragrances: Grapefruit, lemon, mint, cardamom, clove, coriander, cinnamon, and black pepper. These are either oils from plants that stimulate digestion or oils that are spicier and warmer.

Associated number: 10

Associated mantra: RAM

Associated Foods: This Chakra receives energy primarily from yellow-colored foods such as lemons, bananas, pineapples, peppers, wheat and cereal, ginger and turmeric, sunflower seeds, and cheese.

Heart Chakra (4th)

(Sanskrit name: Anahata)

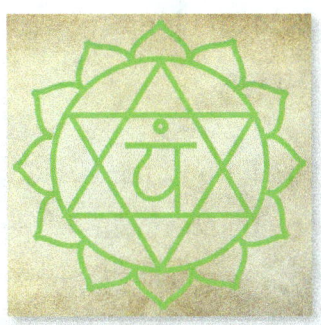

Element: Air

Color: Green

Position: In the center of the chest

Planet: Venus

Characteristics of the well-balanced Chakra: This Chakra represents the place where love and tenderness are born. It is responsible for the balance of our emotions and our openness to life and relationships. The main purpose of this Chakra is the expression of love in all its forms and, when the energy flows correctly, we feel proud, full of pleasure, love, and trust, ready to forgive anyone. It balances the heart and mind, promotes healing, and gives a sense of calm and tranquility. It is the seat of the purest energy and feelings and acts as a bridge toward the spiritual world. When it is well balanced we feel happy and motivated.

Personal qualities related to this Chakra: Unconditioned love, healing, compassion, harmony, transformation, devotion, and sharing.

Which organs is it associated with? Heart, vagus nerve, skin, hands and arms, vertebrae, chest, bronchi and lungs, cardiovascular, respiratory, and immune systems.

What physical problems is it related to? Pain in the back, shoulders, arms, and wrists. Pulmonary problems, bronchial asthma, and cardiovascular diseases. Digestive problems and ulcers. Weak eyesight.

What part of the emotional sphere does it affect? This is the Chakra of love, forgiveness, understanding, and motivation. It influences the emotional sphere that revolves around these feelings and emotions.

Symptoms of a blocked Chakra: There is a strong fear of being alone. There are frequent bursts of anger or feelings of deep bitterness, even unjustified. In love, you tend to be suffocating and morbidly jealous. You feel pervaded by a deep sadness of which you cannot identify the cause and you feel pain because of this. You tend to become dependent on feelings and, in some way, on those around you, and on their judgment. One is afraid to commit, tends to cheat, be dishonest, and be alone.

Unhealthy relationships are a clear example of the blockage of this Chakra.

Possible causes of blockage or imbalance: This Chakra is damaged by some of the most common life experiences. For example, having received little love and care as a child and in the growth phase, for example, from an uncaring parent or parent too focused on himself. More extreme situations in childhood can also be a cause of the blockage, such as physical or emotional trauma. They could also be more recent causes such as having developed wrong ideas and beliefs about love or having undertaken bad behavioral habits that prevent giving and healthily receiving love. Blocking this Chakra are the emotional states related to the sensations of internal emotional pain.

Gems of the Heart Chakra: The main gems of this Chakra are Green Tourmaline and Rose Quartz. It is however in harmony with all the stones of green and pink color such as pink and green agate, jade, aventurine, malachite, emerald, and pink and green zircon.

Associated colors: Green and pink

Associated sense: Touch

Associated fragrances: Lavender, rose geranium, rose, lemon balm, and sweet orange. These are essential oils with softening, comforting, sedative, soothing, harmonious, and revitalizing powers.

Associated number: 12

Associated mantra: YAM

Associated foods: This Chakra draws energy from all green vegetables and those that have a green leafy plant. Especially important for the balance of this Chakra are green tea and herbs such as thyme, basil, and marjoram.

NOTE: Excessive energy flowing through this Chakra can lead to a loss of emotional control and, therefore, to the occurring of the wrong emotions at the wrong time. It is vital to take care of the balance and stability of its energy flow at all times.

Throat Chakra (5th)

(Sanskrit name: Vishuddha)

Element: Ether

Color: Blue

Position: Throat, at the intersection with the clavicle

Planet: Saturn

Characteristics of the well-balanced Chakra: Communication, openness to others, and listening. From this Chakra enters and exits "Prana" (the energy we discussed earlier). It has the task of controlling communication and producing sounds. The produced sounds originate vibrations that put us in tune with the vibrations of the universe. It stimulates creativity and gives mental clarity. Its main purpose is to allow our inner voice to be heard. When it is perfectly balanced, we express ourselves adequately and the words come out with a constant pleasant flow. If the energy flows correctly, we are honest, sincere, and good listeners not only for others but also for ourselves. We listen without judging. Sincerity and honesty are both characteristics of this Chakra and they are both directed toward others and ourselves. When this Chakra is in harmony, we really listen to others, to ourselves, to our thoughts, and to our desires. We create opportunities for ourselves, we develop our creative side, we become part of the world, of its universal rhythm, and we connect to others without being conditioned and crushed by their opinions.

Personal qualities related to this Chakra: Freedom, independence, expression of one's creativity, inspiration, truth, sincerity.

Which organs is it associated with? It mainly affects the metabolic system and the respiratory system with the throat, mouth, vocal cords, trachea, larynx, tonsils, bronchi, and lungs. It also affects the esophagus, cervical vertebrae, and the area of arms, shoulders, and neck.

What physical problems is it related to? You may experience thyroid problems, sore throats and chronic infections, discomfort and tension in the neck and shoulders, pain in the ear or in the area of the jaws and jaws, and dizziness and poor balance.

What part of the emotional sphere does it affect? It influences the sphere of giving voice to our emotions without fear and how this allows us to connect to others, to become part of the world, and of its rhythm. This Chakra also influences our creative side, helping us to channel our energies in the best possible way.

Symptoms of a blocked Chakra: We fail to communicate and tend to keep everything inside, including the emotions that we cannot express. We begin to reduce our contact with others, we fear new friendships, and become distrustful as if others are always ignoring our own interests. This often causes us to become manipulative towards others, even unconsciously. We become increasingly lazy, without self-esteem, and with a tendency to fall into immobility.

Possible causes of blockage or imbalance: The blockage or imbalance usually occurs when a person continues to lie to himself and to others. It also occurs when there is a lack of honesty in behaviors and attitudes, both to the detriment of oneself and others.

Gems of Throat Chakra: The main stone of this Chakra is Aquamarine. It is, however, in harmony and resonance with all blue and light blue stones: Sapphire, blue zircon, and turquoise.

Associated colors: Light blue and blue

Associated sense: Hearing

Associated fragrances: Eucalyptus, sage, bergamot, verbena, chamomile, and tea tree. These are essential oils with soothing, harmonizing power, and a balsamic effect.

Associated number: 16

Associated mantra: HAM

Associated foods: Since there are no blue foods in nature, it is difficult to energize this Chakra with food. Water, however, is important for its balance and with it all the drinks that can be made from it, such as juices, teas, infusions, and herbal teas. Algae, which grow in water, are very useful to energize this Chakra, and they are delicious to prepare your dishes.

NOTE: If the flow of energy through this Chakra is too intense, there is a risk of speaking too aggressively, and showing excessive superiority. You develop a tendency to talk too much, too fast, and always interrupt others. For this reason, it is fundamental to keep the flow of this Chakra balanced and constant at all times.

Third Eye Chakra (6th)

(Sanskrit Name: Ajna)

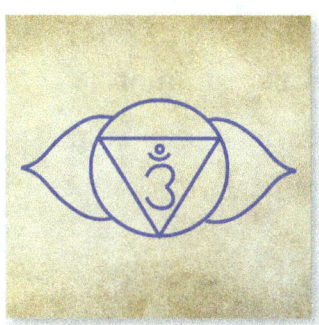

Element: Light

Color: Indigo

Position: Between the eyebrows

Planet: Jupiter

Characteristics of the well-balanced Chakra: Awareness is the main characteristic of the sixth Chakra. The purpose of this Chakra is to understand the bigger picture in every area. It is often associated with the acquisition of supernatural powers because the spiritual sight that it gives us, allows us to see things that escape ordinary people. This Chakra allows us to have a clear vision of what is around us, but also of what is within us. It makes us develop a strong intuition, almost always right, and deals with our communication with the subconscious, where our deepest motivations lie. It allows us to become aware of ourselves, who we really are, what we really need, and what our reality is. Thanks to the sixth Chakra, we can be centered in the here and now, we can see beyond appearances, and disengage ourselves from material possessions, the fear of death, and other paralyzing phobias. It protects us from outside influences, opens us up to and facilitates change. It helps us to develop freedom of thought and inspiration, often expressed through art forms. It makes us focused, determined, and have a clear idea of what is real, and what is illusory.

Personal qualities related to this Chakra: Intuition, clairvoyance, imagination, projection of the will, and mental peace.

Which organs is it associated with? Nose, forehead, temples, ears, left eye, nervous system, cerebellum, marrow, and hormonal system.

What physical problems is it related to? Problems of sight, hearing, sinusitis, and also hormonal dysfunctions are frequent and linked to imbalances in this Chakra.

What part of the emotional sphere does it influence? It is a Chakra strongly linked to mood, fears, and the distinction between dreams and reality.

Symptoms of a blocked Chakra: When this Chakra is blocked, unmotivated mood swings are frequent. You are not able to keep your fears under control. You often find yourself lost in a fantasy world, lost in continuous daydreams. Being the Chakra of our Third Eye, if a veil covers the eye (it blocks the eye), we are not able to see beyond appearances, and we see in a blurred way. For this reason, another symptom of the blockage is the loss of intuition, which makes us close in on ourselves because we can no longer see anything around us, neither material nor spiritual. We tend to worry about any triviality and we are afraid of things that probably will never happen. Nervousness and insomnia are common. So are feelings of apathy, distrust, depression, and a sense of worthlessness. Often accompanying these feelings is the sensation of no longer having feelings because you can't see or recognize them. This is what causes the tendency to live in the world of dreams, so as not to see a surrounding reality that we do not like.

Possible causes of blockage or imbalance: This Chakra is usually blocked when we tend to live in the world of dreams, far away from reality, without ever doing anything to make these dreams come true, and allowing them to remain only fantasies.

Gems of Third Eye Chakra: The main stone of this Chakra is Amethyst. It is in resonance with all purple stones which are powerful in promoting mental processes and concentration. The most popular purple stones are purple zircon, lapis lazuli, calcite, and fluorite.

Associated colors: Indigo and violet

Associated sense: Sixth sense

Associated fragrance: Artemisia, mint, rosemary, lavender, star anise, thyme, and neroli. These are essential oils that stimulate the intellectual and intuitive side, and send messages of a subtle nature.

Associated number: 2

Mantra: AUM

Associated foods: To energize this Chakra you need foods and drinks that stimulate mental energy, such as tea and coffee, for example. Indigo fruits and vegetables, such as eggplant, berries, and grapes, are also good. A good alternative is given by plants with indigo flowers such as rosemary, or juniper, for infusions, and to flavor your dishes.

NOTE: The flow of energy in this Chakra must be balanced and constant because in case of excessive flow you may experience feelings of continuous distraction, and impatience, and you may bring to an access your sense of ambition. When excess of flow in the energy of this Chakra occurs, the person does not take responsibility, tends to exalts his own talents too much, and tends to unload his own faults and errors onto others.

Crown Chakra (7th)

(Sanskrit Name: Sahasrara)

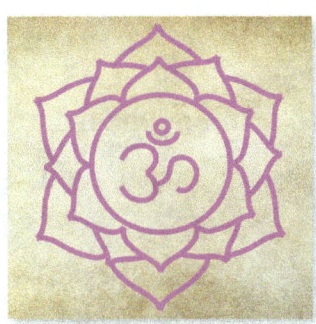

Element: Time and Space

Color: Violet

Position: On the top of the head

Planet: Neptune

Characteristics of the well-balanced Chakra: The seventh Chakra is the center of spirituality, through which we can channel cosmic energy. It gives us purity, helps us to channel our light, makes us creative, and pushes us to constantly improve. It teaches us to trust our inner voice because we have arrived at a very deep knowledge and awareness of ourselves, an almost transcendental knowledge. It makes us skilled observers, able to notice with awareness what is happening around us. The past does not influence us in any way, we have not forgotten it, it simply does not influence us anymore because we have taken responsibility for our mistakes, and we have overcome the traumas. Our thinking is clean and we can recognize our merits as well because we are free from mental impositions. The main purpose of this Chakra is to make us live consciously.

Personal qualities related to this Chakra: Bliss, enlightenment, understanding, universal awareness, and divine wisdom.

Which organs is it associated with? The central nervous system, cerebral cortex, right eye, brain, and skull.

What physical problems is it related to? Among the most frequent physical symptoms are depression, sensitivity to light, and learning difficulties.

What part of the emotional sphere does it influence? This Chakra influences, from the emotional point of view, the understanding both of oneself and of others. In fact, when this Chakra is blocked or unbalanced this understanding is lost, causing the problems discussed below.

Symptoms of a blocked Chakra: When this Chakra is blocked, one tends to be rigid, superficial, unsatisfied, and too attached to material things. High fear of death is very common because it is perceived as the end of everything. We lose sight of the good things in life and feel estranged from everything around us. Often there is a strong attachment to what you have, caused by the thought of not deserving anything else, and for this reason, you constantly belittle yourself.

Possible causes of blockage or imbalance: Usually this Chakra is blocked when we manifest too strong an attachment to the material and earthly world, for example, an excessive attachment to work, home, or people. These excessive sensations of attachment and belonging lead to blocks and imbalances.

Gems of the Crown Chakra: The main stone of this Chakra is the rock crystal (hyaline quartz), which helps to overcome personal problems, and makes us deepen our knowledge of ourselves. This Chakra also resonates with white or transparent stones such as diamond, colorless zircon, iridescent opal, and white agate.

Associated colors: White (because it encloses all colors), transparent and purple

Associated sense: No physical sense

Associated fragrances: Rose, jasmine, sandalwood, lavender, myrrh, and olibanum. These are essential oils with a persistent fragrance that stimulate the connection with the divine and spiritual development.

Associated number: 1000

Associated mantra: OM

Associated Foods: This Chakra benefits from foods and drinks with detoxifying and purifying effects, since it is dealing with less physical energy than the other Chakras. Lotus and lavender are great for balancing and energizing it.

NOTE: Excessive functioning of this Chakra leads to a strong distraction in achieving your goals. If you do not quickly achieve what you want, you tend to give up and this leads you to never achieve anything. Its correct flow in a balanced way is, therefore, fundamental to living a fulfilling and satisfying life.

How to Balance and Heal Your Chakras

In the previous chapter, we looked in detail at each of the 7 main Chakras. At this point, you should have a very clear picture of the sphere of interest of each Chakra and some of the elements that can influence it positively or negatively. For example, now you should be able to recognize what negative behaviors can block the energy flow of a certain Chakra, and also choose what color, stone, or essence can help to heal a certain Chakra, and to make its energy flow correctly. Also, with the knowledge gained, you should be able to identify which ones are your blocked or unbalanced Chakras, so you can start working toward healing them. The section dedicated to the symptoms in each Chakra is the main tool for your diagnosis. If you recognize your current situation in any of the emotional, mental, or physical symptoms described then you know you need to intervene in the Chakra that originates those symptoms. In the next few pages, we will look at the various options available to you to open, unlock, and heal your Chakras. Most options are DIY, for others you might need a little help but you will surely find one or more options suitable for you.

First, however, I would like to bring your attention to an important point: unlocking the Chakras is not permanent. It is an ongoing process. After unlocking a Chakra, a lack of energy may occur, causing a new closure, or an imbalance in the energy flow with the consequent recurrence of related problems. Your goal must, therefore, be to completely avoid blockages and imbalances, and keep the energy flow well and balanced constantly. To do this, you need to take constant care of each one of your Chakras. Always pay attention to symptoms that indicate a lack of energy flow or a potential blockage, try to listen to yourself, and keep an eye and try to notice the signals of your body because this simple step of analysis and awareness will be your first ally in the path for healing Chakras, and to improve your everyday life.

My advice is to create your own regular routine of total care to balance your Chakras so that you can enjoy constant benefits mentally, physically, spiritually, and emotionally. Another piece of advice I would like to give you is to work on all of your Chakras regularly, especially if you are in doubt about which of the 7 Chakras needs the most immediate or major intervention. You may need, especially in the beginning, to work with particular intensity on only one of them at a time, but then you should focus on balancing all 7 to improve your overall mental, physical, spiritual, and emotional health.

There are mainly 7 methods for healing and balancing your Chakras and we will cover them throughout the book. We will see in detail how each technique applies to the different

Chakras, in the meantime, I list below what these methods are, so you can start to get an idea.

Here are the 7 techniques with which you can heal. open and balance your Chakras:

1. Affirmations and Mantra Repetition

2. Meditation

3. Yoga

4. Massage

5. Chromotherapy

6. Crystal Therapy

7. Therapy with Essential Oils

We'll break them all down individually in the next pages and we'll also discuss how, and whether to combine them for maximum results. We'll also discuss the ones you can easily apply on your own and the ones you may need professional support for.

Affirmations and Mantras

I have chosen to begin with Mantras and Affirmations because they are one of the easiest methods to balance the Chakras and, above all, it is a method that you can easily apply on your own, without interfering too much with your everyday habits. Unfortunately, they may not be completely effective on their own, especially in case of imbalances or blockages that are too pronounced, but they help to keep the Chakras in optimal balance if they are practiced regularely (it would be ideal to make them part of a routine, as I suggested before).

My suggestion is to practice this method every day, for a few minutes, focusing each day on a different Chakra. What you have to do is to repeat aloud the affirmation or the specific Mantra of a certain Chakra. No phrase or mantra has an effect on all Chakras at the same time and, for this reason, I suggested that you focus on a Chakra for each day of the week (it is very convenient since there are 7 days and 7 Chakras).

As for the affirmations, I suggest you repeat them out loud while looking in the mirror. Ideally, you should practice these repetitions for a few minutes twice a day, possibly in the morning just after getting up, and in the evening before going to bed. This positive dialogue with yourself brings truly incredible results.

For Mantras, on the other hand, I recommend doing this whenever you have a few free minutes where you can sit in a relaxed pose, with your eyes closed. You will have to pronounce them aloud and the vibrations of those sounds will make you vibrate in tune with the energy of the Chakra you are working on.

In the section where I described the individual Chakras, I listed the Mantra associated with each one but I will list them in the chart below for your convenience. Subsequently, I will list both in detail and in a similar chart the affirmation related to each Chakra, and all my suggestions to optimize the application.

Mantras

Chakra	Mantra
1º Chakra - Root	LAM
2º Chakra - Sacral	VAM
3º Chakra - Solar Plexus	RAM
4º Chakra - Heart	YAM
5º Chakra - Throat	HAM
6º Chakra - Third Eye	AUM
7º Chakra - Crown	OM

Affirmations

I. Root Chakra

The main affirmation related to this Chakra is:

I AM

This affirmation is sufficient to balance the Chakra, but for many, it does not work because they cannot identify with it as it is. Therefore it is often necessary to make the phrase more complete and specific. For example, for many it is useful to say that you are beautiful on a mental or physical level, for others to be safe and have everything you need, for others still to be centered, to be happy, to be in your body and be yourself, and even to be connected to the nature that surrounds you.

"I AM BEAUTIFUL"

"I AM SAFE AND HAVE EVERYTHING I NEED"

"I AM CENTERED AND ROOTED"

"I AM HAPPY TO BE IN MY BODY"

"I AM CONTENT TO BE MYSELF"

"I AM CONNECTED TO NATURE"

II. Sacral Chakra

The main affirmation related to this Chakra is:

I FEEL

This affirmation is about our ability to feel sensations and experience them. As for the previous affirmation, the main sentence "I feel" is sufficient but for many people, it works better to have more complete sentences.

For example:

"I FEEL JOY AND HAPPINESS"

"I FEEL PLEASURE"

"I FEEL CREATIVE"

"I FEEL FULL OF JOY"

"I FEEL SENSUAL AND EMBRACE MY SEXUALITY"

"I FEEL LIKE HONORING MY DESIRES"

"I FEEL PLAYFUL AND SPONTANEOUS"

"I FEEL I DESERVE TO ENJOY LIFE"

"I FEEL HEALTHY"

"I HAVE HEALTHY FEELINGS"

"I FEEL ALIVE AND FACE THE WORLD WITHOUT FEAR"

III. Solar Plexus Chakra

The main affirmation related to this Chakra is:

I DO

You can practice it as it is, or create phrases if you feel more comfortable with them. The affirmations of this Chakra are mainly about action and doing.

For example:

"I ACT WITH COURAGE"

"I CARRY OUT MY TASKS EASILY"

"I HONOR MYSELF"

"I ACT WITH POWER"

"MY POTENTIAL IS UNLIMITED"

"I AM RESPONSIBLE FOR THE ACTIONS IN MY LIFE"

IV. Heart Chakra

The main affirmation related to this Chakra is:

I LOVE

For most people, it is easy to recognize this affirmation as their own and practice it easily as it is. However, it can be enriched by many nuances and you can choose those that best suit you if you prefer them to the main affirmation.

For example:

"I LOVE MYSELF AND OTHERS"

"I AM AN EXPRESSION OF LOVE"

"I DESERVE TO BE LOVED"

"I FORGIVE MYSELF AND OTHERS"

"I FOLLOW THE VOICE OF MY HEART"

"I AM LOVED"

"I ACT WITH LOVE"

"I AM FULL OF LOVE"

V. Throat Chakra

The main affirmation related to this Chakra is:

I SAY

The affirmations linked to this Chakra are associated with speaking and communicating. The main affirmation can be practiced as it is, or you can use the formula "I SPEAK". All for all the previous affirmations, in this case as well you can create richer and more complete affirmations, if they make more sense to you, and make your practice easier.

For example:

"I HEAR AND SPEAK THE TRUTH"

"MY VOICE IS IMPORTANT"

"I SPEAK AND MY WORDS EXPRESS INTEGRITY"

"I SPEAK OPENLY AND HONESTLY AND LIVE AN AUTHENTIC LIFE"

"I RECEIVE AND COMMUNICATE AN IMPORTANT MESSAGE"

"I SPEAK HONEST, TRUE, AND SINCERE WORDS"

VI. Third Eye Chakra

The main affirmation related to this Chakra is:

I SEE

The affirmation of this Chakra is linked to both physical and spiritual sight. The main affirmation is easy to practice for most people and very powerful. However, I list a series of more articulated or complete affirmations, which can give you ideas if you need a full sentence to practice better.

For example:

"I SEE CLEARLY"

"I CAN SEE INTO MYSELF AND OTHERS, AND I AM INTUITIVE"

"I THINK AND I SEE MY THOUGHTS CLEARLY"

"I SEE CLEARLY WHEN I DECIDE AND I TRUST MY DECISIONS"

"I SEE AND THIS EXPANDS MY AWARENESS"

"I BELIEVE IN MY INTUITION AND I TRUST IT"

VII. Crown Chakra

The main affirmation related to this Chakra is:

I UNDERSTAND

The affirmation of this Chakra is linked to the supreme understanding, enlightenment, and comprehension of the all world in its spirituality. The main affirmation can be easily practiced as it is. Even in its simplicity, it contains an incredible strength. It can be varied to "I KNOW" or "I UNDERSTAND" if you feel these phrases are more akin to you. Finally, understanding can be declined in an infinite number of nuances and you may prefer a more articulate statement.

For example:

"I KNOW THAT I AM A DIVINE BEING"

"I KNOW I AM A SPIRITUAL BEING"

"I UNDERSTAND THAT I AM ONE WITH THE WHOLE"

"I KNOW THAT I AM INFINITE AND WITHOUT BOUNDARIES"

"I UNDERSTAND AND I AM AT PEACE"

"I AM OPEN TO UNDERSTANDING AND ENLIGHTENMENT"

Below you can find the resuming chart I promised with the main affirmation of each Chakra. It can be useful to you, just as much as the one I made about the Mantras at the beginning of the chapter. I used to make these little charts for myself when I was just starting my healing journey. I kept a picture of them on my phone and some printed copies in my bag, or in my purse because it took me a little while to learn them by heart. Always having a copy with me helped me a lot in difficult times when I need to practice but I could remember what. You could do this too, it would certainly come in handy and make things a lot easier. When you are starting on a new habit, the easier the better, trust me on this.

Chakra	Mantra
1º Chakra - Root	I AM
2º Chakra - Sacral	I FEEL
3º Chakra - Solar Plexus	I DO
4º Chakra - Heart	I LOVE
5º Chakra - Throat	I SAY
6º Chakra - Third Eye	I SEE
7º Chakra - Crown	I UNDERSTAND

Meditation

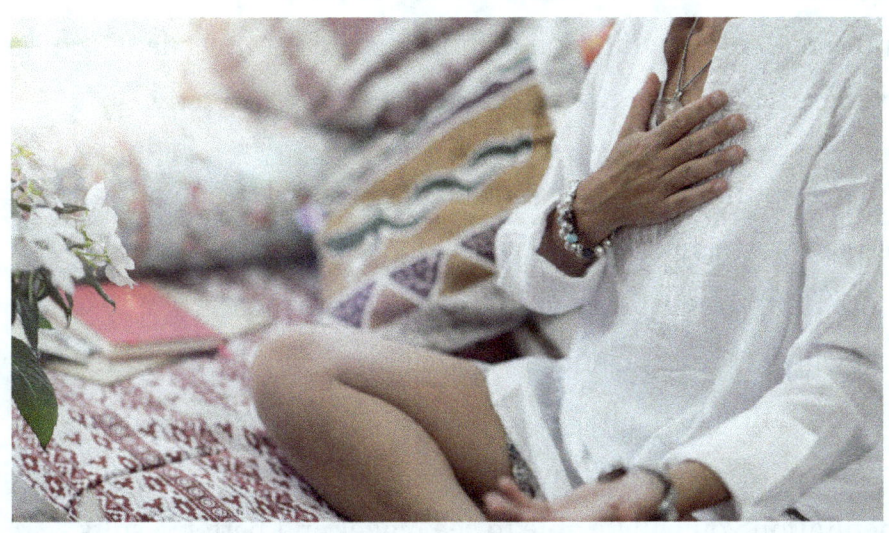

Meditation helps us to awaken the energy of our body and, for this reason, is an excellent cure for our closed, blocked, or unbalanced Chakras. Meditation, like Mantras and affirmations, is a method that you can apply with total autonomy. This makes it very useful and valuable because you can practice it whenever you want and feel the need for it. You don't depend on the help of others to practice it and that's great because, if you live on a busy schedule, you can just arrange the opportunity to practice during a coffee or lunch break.

Many people are afraid of the idea of meditating because they believe they are not able to do it. In truth, it's very easy! To start meditating you just need to let your thoughts free to flow or hold one thought and let all the others flow away from your head. Meditating for the Chakras does not require particularly high or transcendental meditation techniques, just simple visualization exercises, appropriate music, and breathing correctly.

So, meditating for the Chakras is really simple and you can refine your technique with repetition and practice. Also, the more time you dedicate to this activity, the greater the results you will get. You can start by dedicating just a few minutes a day to meditation to begin to see the first positive changes and improvements. As you invest more time in the activity of meditation you will be able to see bigger and better results.

You can meditate on a single Chakra, or you can work on all of them simultaneously, according to your needs and requirements. This makes this practice even greater because it allows you to take care of all your Chakras at one time.

You could, or rather you should create a meditation corner. You should choose a quiet place just for yourself, possibly in your house. You should decorate your meditation space with cushions and mats to be comfortable, and surround yourself with objects, colors, stones, and essences to further stimulate your Chakras. (We will talk more about this further stimulation of your Chakras later).

Now let's look at the strongest but simplest meditation techniques that you can start applying immediately to heal, unblock, and balance your Chakras.

Color Meditation

The color meditation is the simplest Chakra meditation. Even if it is so simple it has a great impact on your Chakras' health.

Let's see how to practice it step-by-step.

1. First of all, you will need to find a quiet place where you feel comfortable or simply go to your meditation corner if you have organized one. You will have to sit in a comfortable position and I recommend wearing comfortable clothes to be as comfortable as possible. It would be ideal to have a straight back so that all the Chakras are aligned during the meditation.

2. Now close your eyes. Breath with your nose. Concentrate on your breathing for a few minutes and take deep breaths in a single air flux. Inhale for about 4 seconds and exhale all the air you let in taking exactly the same amount of time, 4 seconds. Keep breathing in this way during all the practice.

3. Starting from the lowest Chakra, visualize the color of that Chakra, feel pervaded by the energy of that color,

and keep this thought and this sensation for at least 4 minutes, during which the color inside you should become brighter and brighter.

4. Use your breath to give a rhythm to your meditation, every time you inspire the color pervades you more and becomes more intense and brilliant.

5. After at least 4 minutes you can move on to the next color, and repeat the sequence from step 3 until you have covered the entire color spectrum of your 7 Chakras. When you are finished, wait a few seconds then slowly open your eyes.

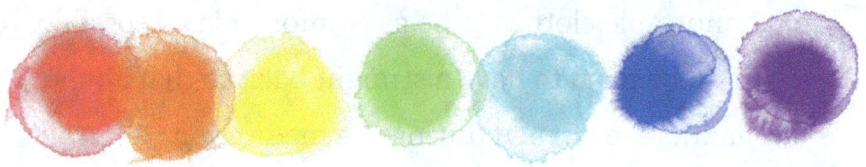

You can practice this meditation in different ways:

- You can go through all 7 Chakra colors. This is useful if you are working on maintaining the balance of all the Chakras.

- You can work on one Chakra at a time. If you feel a particular pleasure in working on one color, it may be that that particular color needs more attention, so you could devote yourself only to it, and stay on it for the whole meditation time. The same if you already know you have to work on a particular Chakra, you will devote the entire meditation to its color.

- If you only have small spaces of time to dedicate to meditation, that's fine too. It would be ideal to be able to do at least 5 minutes at a time, several times a day if you can. Choose, according to your needs, whether to practice a different color at each session or to focus on the same color each time.

- I summarized, in the chart below, the color of each Chakra for your convenience, in case you haven't memorized them yet. I already explained the bests you can do with these charts.

Chakra	Color
1º Chakra - Root	RED
2º Chakra - Sacral	ORANGE
3º Chakra - Solar Plexus	YELLOW
4º Chakra - Heart	GREEN
5º Chakra - Throat	LIGHT BLUE
6º Chakra - Third Eye	INDIGO
7º Chakra - Crown	VIOLET

The 7 Chakras' Meditation

The 7 Chakras' meditation is a little more articulated than the previous one and is extremely powerful. Let's see together, step-by-step, how to practice it in the most correct and effective way:

1. You will need to find a quiet place where you feel comfortable or simply go to your meditation corner. You will need to sit in a comfortable position and I recommend wearing comfortable clothes to be as comfortable as possible and in a general condition of easiness. It would be ideal to sit with a straight back so that all the Chakras are aligned during the meditation. Close your eyes.

2. Breath with your nose. Concentrate on your breathing for a few minutes and take deep breaths in a single air flux. Inhale for about 4 seconds and exhale all the air you let in taking exactly the same amount of time, 4 seconds. Keep breathing in this way during all the practice.

3. After about a minute or two of concentrating on breathing, you should begin to focus on every part of your body, starting from your head down to your feet. You will need to relax each part of your body that you focus on. Try to see in your mind's eye every single muscle that relaxes as you focus on it: your forehead

flattening, your lips stretching, your neck releasing the tension, and so on down to your toes. This is important because you don't want to be too tense or stiff in your sitting position.

4. Now let's move on to breathing. You will have to focus your attention on your breathing: inhale and exhale, in and out. You don't have to force it in any way, just keep focusing your attention on it and you will see that it will slowly become deeper and deeper and more regular. While you are putting air into your lungs, try to visualize it. Try to see the air that enters your lungs, spreads through the blood, enters the muscles, and every cell in your body. When you let the air out, visualize the air coming out of your body taking with it all the toxins and garbage that clog your body. Remember always to breathe through your nose so that fewer impurities enter your body.

5. When you feel your breath proceeding naturally deeply and regularly, you should turn your concentration to your heartbeat. Visualize your heart beating and, at each pulse, moves your blood to reach every part of your body. When the blood reaches every part of your body all those parts enter in harmony and communication with each other. Travel with your blood, reach every part of your

body and feel this wonderful living organism full of strength and energy. Each breath makes your heart beat and brings your body to life.

6. Now imagine that with each breath you take, you let energy into your body, an energy that flows into you along with the air and pervades you with a life force. Create a clear image in your mind. See this energy flowing into your body, see your body absorbing the energy, and becoming stronger. It is a gradual process, with each breath your body becomes stronger and more enlightened by this wonderful energy until your body will glow with a clear and brilliant halo. Build a clear picture of this halo in your mind.

7. Now, you have to channel this energy into each Chakra. As always, you will have to start from the lowest Chakra, the Root, and gradually move upward until you reach the Crown. You will have to visualize your Chakra as a small luminous sphere that rotates clockwise. With each breath, the sphere receives energy and becomes stronger and brighter. You must repeat this visualization for each Chakra until the one you are focused on is full of vital energy. It takes time and some Chakras will take longer than others. When a Chakra takes longer to feel full of energy is because that particular Chakra needs more care

than another. Your mind knows this and guides you through the healing process. In this phase, it is important to move in an orderly way from the bottom to the top without haste, dedicating to each Chakra the time it needs. This is because each Chakra is connected to the one above it and by practicing in the correct we can maintain a perfect balance.

8. Once you have concluded the visualization process for each of the 7 Chakras, take a few seconds, and then slowly open your eyes. Before getting up, I suggest you take a few minutes to try to understand how you feel physically, mentally, spiritually, and emotionally. This moment of analysis is very important both because you will enjoy the pleasant sensations that meditation leaves you and because it will serve as a parameter. Each time you stop to analyze your meditation, you will find that you feel better than the previous time in at least one of the four areas but more often in all four at the same time. You'll feel better physically, mentally, spiritually, and emotionally.

This meditation, being a bit more structured, takes at least half an hour to practice. Some speak of completing it in a quarter of an hour, I personally never managed to complete it in such a short time. My advice is not to rush it and if you already know that you don't have at least thirty minutes, you could fall back on the color meditation which is a good faster option.

Meditating on a single Chakra

It is also possible to concentrate the meditation on a single Chakra if instead of creating a general balance we need to quickly heal a particularly suffering Chakra.

The preparation is the same as described in steps 1 through 6 of the "7 Chakras' Meditation". In step 7, instead of gradually going through all 7 Chakras from bottom to top, you will concentrate only and exclusively on the Chakra you need to quickly heal.

You will have to channel the energy generated in the first 6 steps into the Chakra you are working on. All your concentration will have to be on it. Visualize your small luminous sphere that rotates clockwise, with each breath the sphere receives energy and becomes stronger and brighter. You will have to dedicate to this Chakra all the time it needs and repeat the process daily until you feel you have healed it.

In this regard, never skip the last step, the one of analysis, and understanding because only through it you can understand how you feel physically, mentally, spiritually, and emotionally after each meditation.

The average time required by the meditation on a single Chakra is at least 10-15 minutes, a time easier to carve out than the 30 minutes of the complete 7 Chakras' meditation. One thing that over time I have found very useful is to practice the complete sequence of the 7 Chakras' meditation once a week and then practice the single Chakra meditation once a day for the next 7 days, addressing the Chakras in order from lowest to highest. This is a suggestion for those with limited time, but I think it will come in handy as you build your Chakras' healing routine. I have learned from personal experience that you need to find the best way to fit these important moments into your hectic daily life, and organizing a routine that takes into account the time you have available daily is essential. If you don't create your own Chakra healing routine, you won't benefit from it in the end, and this book will have been nothing more than a pleasant read.

By consistently practicing Chakras' meditation, in any of its variations, you will see incredible results in your daily life, on all levels: in your professional life, in your personal and emotional life, and even in your health. You will gain an inner wholeness and lucidity that will give you noticeable results on a physical, mental, spiritual, and emotional level.

Earth's Meditation

A meditation that has always made me feel very good when I needed to gain energy to balance my Chakras is the one called "Earth's meditation".

This form of meditation consists exactly of the first 6 steps of the 7 Chakras' meditation with two fundamental differences. First, it should not be practiced indoors but outdoors, sitting in close contact with Mother Earth (hence its name). So, eyes closed, back straight, but sitting in a quiet corner in the middle of nature: in a park, a forest, near a stream, on the shore of a lake, or any other place of natural wonder where you feel good and comfortable.

Second, when you have accumulated all the energy through the 6 steps, you will not need to focus on the Chakras, but you will need to stay focused on the life force that is coming to you from nature and Mother Earth. You will have to continue to focus on your breathing, on this life force that grows inside you, pervades you every time you inhale, and expels negative energy and toxins every time you exhale.

It is impossible to estimate a time for this meditation because you merge so much with the nature around you that you could practice it for hours without noticing the passage of time. Of course, it is not so easy to practice it because it is not easy to find quiet corners of unspoiled nature unless you are lucky enough to live in the countryside outside the city.

I invite you, however, to seek out these corners and these moments from time to time because the well-being that this meditation can give you is impossible to describe in words. For me, it has always been a bit like recharging my personal batteries with energy that my Chakras will channel and make flow.

Again, I invite you not to forget point 8. Open your eyes when you have finished your meditation, but before you get up, take all the time you need to understand how you feel physically, mentally, spiritually, and emotionally, and to fully enjoy that wonderful feeling of well-being that I am sure will pervade you.

In the beginning, it will probably feel a little strange to meditate on your Chakras, especially if you have never meditated before in your life but with time and practice it will become as natural as breathing and you won't be able to do without because it will make you feel infinitely good on every level.

Tricks for Chakra Meditation

There are small elements that you can implement during your meditation to favor the energy of a Chakra rather than another, or even make the energy of individual Chakras more effective. Let's see what they are for every single Chakra and how to use them to your advantage:

- **1st Chakra:** To release tension and get even better results when meditating for this Chakra, the ideal would be to meditate while sitting on the ground. Not necessarily outdoors, although that would be even better. This is because it is the Root Chakra, the root that sinks into Mother Earth and the earth is its element.

- **2nd Chakra:** The Sacral Chakra is strongly linked to the element of water. If you meditate for this Chakra you could put the sound of waves, flowing, or gurgling water in the background to make the meditation more powerful. You could also meditate sitting in the bathtub, partially immersed in the water.

- **3rd Chakra:** If you meditate for the Solar Plexus Chakra, the fundamental element to make the meditation more effective is silence. It is characteristic of this Chakra to maintain attention, calm, and silence. Using these three elements during your meditation is very useful for the 3rd

Chakra. Silence itself could be a form of meditation for the health of this Chakra.

- **4th Chakra:** The element of the heart Chakra is air and breathing is the fundamental element if you meditate for this Chakra. You have learned in this chapter the importance of breathing during meditation, importance that becomes even greater when you meditate for the fourth Chakra.

- **5th Chakra:** For the Throat Chakra, words are a magical instrument whose vibrations put us in tune with the universe. To make the meditation for this Chakra more intense, you could repeat a mantra while meditating, or chant.

- **6th Chakra:** The last two Chakras are much more connected to spirituality, so to favor them during meditation you will have to do things less related to the physical world. To better meditate on the Third Eye Chakra you will have to free your mind from the thoughts that continue to crowd it and try to acquire a clearer inner vision.

- **7th Chakra:** To intensify the meditation for the Crown Chakra you will have to expand your connection with the universal energy and focus deeply on your spirituality and on the awareness that you are a spiritual being in a physical body.

Yoga

At this point, we can safely say that the Chakras are a fundamental tool to take care of to maintain ourselves and our bodies in good health at all levels. From this point of view, we can say that yoga is a kind of architect that allows us to implement this project of taking care of ourselves. There are specific positions that allow us to balance or unlock every Chakra.

Although it is a very effective method, you may not be able to use it in total autonomy. If you have had previous experience with yoga and have learned the fundamentals you won't experience any problems. If, however, you are completely new to this discipline, it would be ideal to take a few lessons with an experienced teacher to learn the basics that will allow you to proceed on your own. There are also many good and useful online yoga academies. They give you the chance to attend yoga classes according to your schedule. It is very important to have these basics because mistakes in practice or posture could lead to physical damage, easily avoidable with the advice of an expert. If, however, you already know the basics, many positions can help you unlock your Chakras. Let's see 7 of them, one for each Chakra:

1st Chakra - Root: *Position Of The Tree* (Vrksasana)

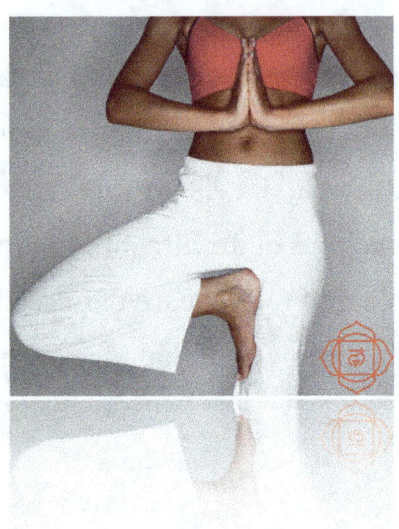

2nd Chakra - Sacral: *Position Of The Goddess* (Deviasana)

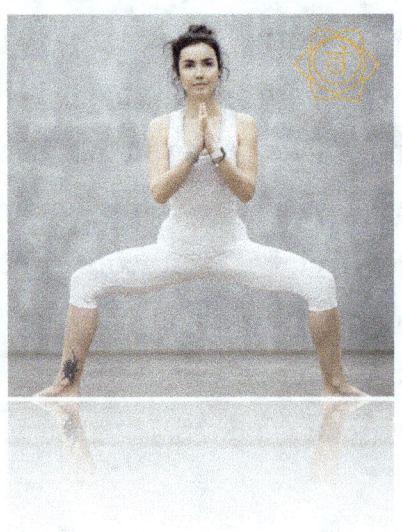

3rd Chakra - Solar Plexus: Position Of The Boat (Navasana)

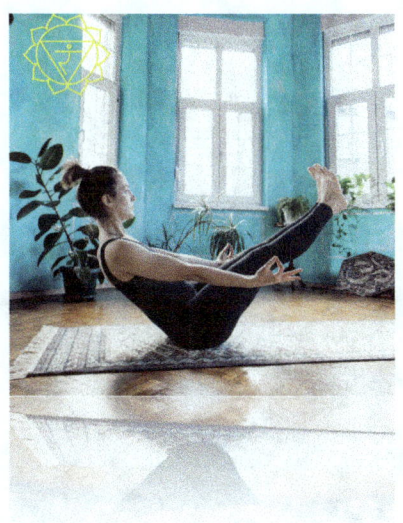

4th Chakra - Heart: Position Of The Camel (Ustrasana)

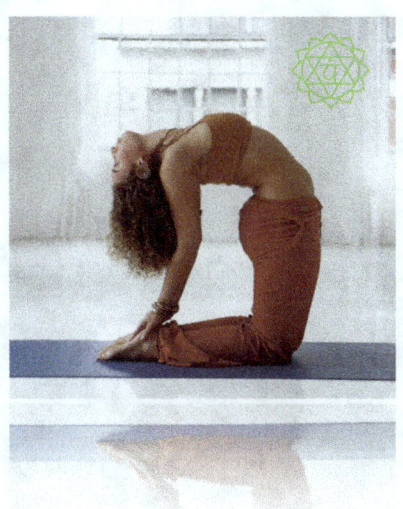

5th Chakra - Throat: Position Of The Candle With Support (Salamba Sarvangasana)

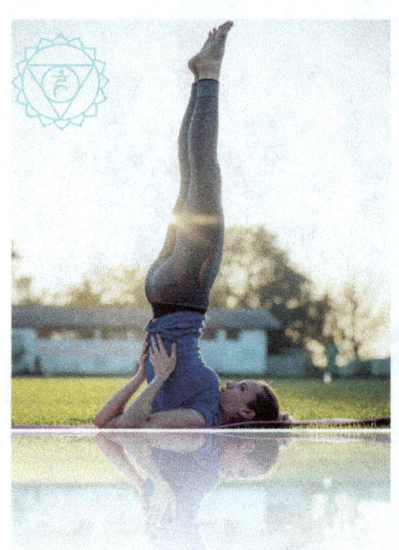

6th Chakra - Third Eye: Comfortable Position (Sukhasana)

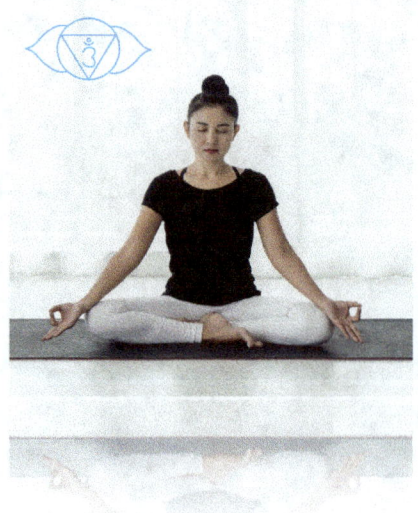

7th Chakra - Crown: Corpse Position (Savasana)

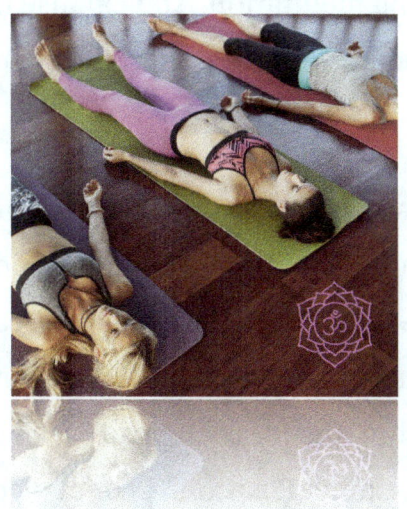

You can do the sequence in full and in order, as always from the bottom Chakra up, or you can focus on the Chakra you are working on. You can also work on two or three Chakras only. In this case, pick the yoga poses of each Chakra you are working on to build your yoga sequence, your choice depends on the areas of your life you are focusing on that require healing.

If during your practice you experience a sense of restlessness that you cannot easily calm or control my advice is to hold the position(s) you are practicing longer. This will help you to be more present and grounded, and to eliminate the sense of restlessness.

Breathing is very important when practicing yoga, just as much as when practicing meditation. You can use the same kind of breathing technique we discussed in the chapter about meditation.

Breath with your nose. Inhale and exhale from a single flux of air. Take 4 seconds every time you inhale and 4 seconds when you exhale. Take long, relaxed, and deep breaths. Remember to breathe even when you are holding a position. To help me with this, I count the breaths for each position I hold. For example, when I hold the "Camel Position" I count 3 complete sequences of breathing before changing position. My exceptions are Sukhasana e Savasana. In Sukhasana I only concentrate on breathing properly, in Savasana I let my body totally relax and I let my breath run freely according to my relaxed condition.

Just so you know, the name of this breathing technique is "Ujjayi Breathing" ("The Winning Breath") and it has one more main characteristic apart from the ones already described. When breathing, you should try to close a little the top part of your throat so that the air stays longer in the top part of your breathing system. In this way, air maintains a longer contact with your mucous membrane rich in blood, which makes the air you breathe a lot warmer, giving your body a relaxed feeling.

Massages

If you have experienced a massage at least once in your life, you know how beneficial it is for your body, your mind, and your. spirit. When you are massaged you feel all the tension in your body melt away, stress leaves you, and you feel in a delightful state of absolute grace for a few days after.

This wonderful practice can be used to help your Chakras, to open them up, and to keep them in balance. Not all Chakras need the same type of massage, in fact, the type of massage varies depending on the Chakra you want to work on and its location.

To get the most out of this practice my advice is to ask an expert, so you can let yourself go completely and enjoy the massage in total relaxation. It is however possible to stimulate some areas of your body with a DIY massage that helps to heal your Chakras.

In the following pages, we will see what area to massage and how so that you can stimulate every Chakra on your own. Still, I suggest you go to an expert whenever possible to fully enjoy this wonderful experience. If you are not used to massaging, at first this practice may make you feel a little awkward. Don't worry, all you need is a little practice, and it will soon become a natural gesture that will amaze you with its simplicity, effectiveness, and great results.

The correct way to massage yourself to stimulate and activate your Chakras' energy is with a few simple slow circular movements in a clockwise direction. When you begin to feel comfortable with those movements and the massage, you can try speeding up the rhythm or increasing the pressure. Find the combination that gives you the most pleasant sensation in each part of your body and practice it for 5 to 10 minutes, daily.

As for the methods I described in the previous chapters, you can practice the massage in two ways. You can go through all your Chakras from the bottom one to the top one or you can work with one in particular at a time. If you have little time to dedicate to this practice but you want to work on all the Chakras, you can focus on one single Chakra per day. If you choose this option, remember to always massage your Chakras' in order starting from the bottom and going upward. For example, start on Monday massaging your body to stimulate energy in the Root Chakra, on Tuesday to stimulate the Sacral Chakra, and so on with the rest of the days of the week.

For massage, just like I suggested for meditation, you should create a quiet corner where you can retreat and practice. Peace, silence, and tranquility will help you to put your body in a relaxed state that will make the massage easier and more effective.

To make your hands flow better on your skin, essential oils are an excellent solution. We will see in the dedicated chapter how you can choose oils whose essence and fragrance help the opening and stimulation of the Chakra you are working on healing.

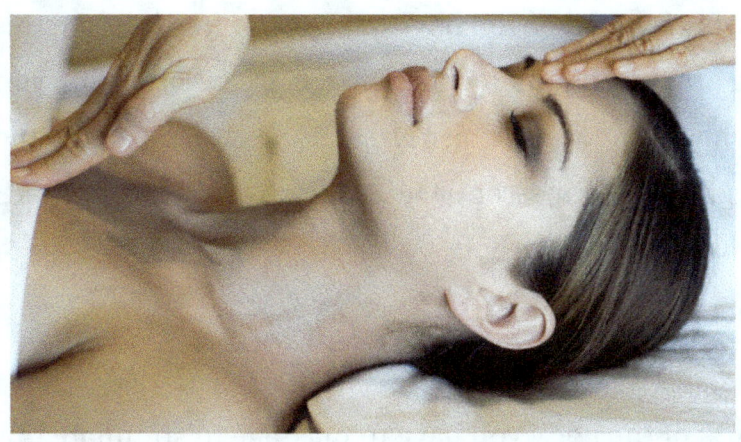

Let's look at the areas to massage for each Chakra:

I. The Root Chakra

The parts of the body you have to massage to stimulate this Chakra are the buttocks, legs, and feet. Dedicate a pleasant massage to this area of your body and let the feeling of well-being radiate throughout your body.

II. The Sacral Chakra

The parts of the body you have to massage to stimulate this Chakra are the area below the navel, the hip area, the lumbar muscles, and the base of the back.

III. The Solar Plexus Chakra

The parts of the body you have to massage to stimulate this Chakra are the abdomen and stomach area. Massaging your stomach with slow clockwise circular movements and hands lightly greased with essential oil will activate an important energy center for your body.

IV. The Heart Chakra

The parts of the body you have to massage to stimulate this Chakra are the chest, shoulders, the beginning of the arm, and the back of the torso. Some areas are difficult to reach, so, do what you can without tugging or straining, and try to keep your muscles relaxed as much as possible. Start with slow circles on the chest, rising just as slowly to the shoulders, then move to the beginning of the arms, and when you move to the back of the torso reach as far as you can without strain or tension.

V. The Throat Chakra

The parts of the body you have to massage to stimulate this Chakra go from the base of the neck, down to the shoulders, going all the way through the neck. Start with light and slow circular rubs from the hairline of the head towards the neck, go down along the back of the neck, and then slowly focus on the muscles that connect the neck to the shoulders. Continue until you feel the desired effect of the tension easing.

VI. The Third Eye Chakra

To stimulate this Chakra we focus on massaging the area of the face, always with slow circular movements. Begin with the temples, forehead, cheeks, cheekbones, and then the jaws. I recommend that you perform this massage with your eyes closed, trying to relax as much as possible. This will help you to better enjoy the feeling of opening your third eye.

VII. The Crown Chakra

This Chakra is stimulated by massaging the head area from the hairline to the entire scalp area. When practiced well and regularly, this massage allows you to enjoy a wonderful feeling of pressure easing, and energy flowing.

A consistent practice of massage will be extremely beneficial in rebalancing and healing your chakras, and you will feel increasingly filled with a new positive and beneficial energy that flows through your body.

Chromotherapy

Chromotherapy is treating the Chakras with the colors of the rainbow.

Our body reacts to colors because each color is a different vibration of energy. According to Ayurvedic medicine, since our body reacts to colors on a physical, emotional, spiritual, and mental level, the 7 colors of the rainbow can rebalance the energy centers of our body, your 7 main Chakras. The principle behind this idea is that life is color and color is life, as opposed to the darkness and gloom of death.

The 7 colors of the rainbow, therefore, restore the balance of our energy centers and influence their health daily. This daily influence manifests itself in an infinite number of ways since most of the objects that surround us are colored. The food you eat, the colors of the clothes you wear, and the colors of the environment in which you live or work influence your Chakras and your energy in every single moment of your life. The influence can be positive or negative. Think about a horrible working place, decorated with colors that make you feel upset or uncomfortable, that's definitely a negative way to use the power of colors in your life. On the other hand, if you use this power with consciousness and a positive purpose, it can bring enormous benefits to the energy flow of your Chakras.

Reflecting light through a prism, we obtain the 7 colors of the rainbow. Those colors show themselves to our eyes in a sequence exactly equivalent to the Chakras' colors, ordered from first to last Chakra.

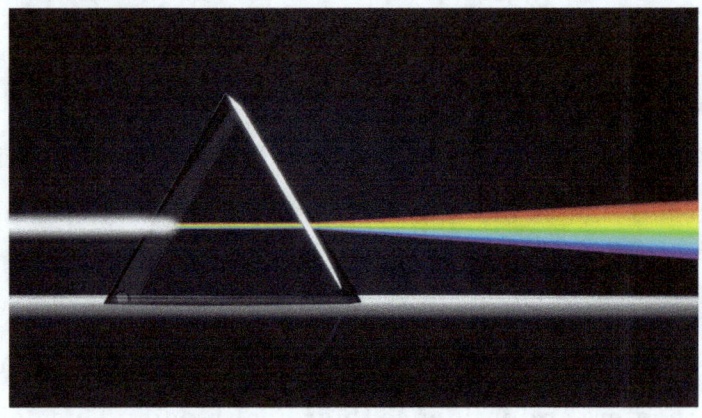

The highest color of the prism corresponds to the first Chakra, the one with the lowest position on the spine. Going down in the colors' sequence of the prism, we go up with the position of the Chakras along the spine.

So:

First Chakra: *Mūlādhāracakra* = Red

Second Chakra: *Svādhisthānacakra* = Orange

Third Chakra: *Manipura* = Yellow

Fourth Chakra: *Anahata* = Green

Fifth Chakra: *Vishudda* = Blue

Sixth Chakra: *Ajna* = Indigo Blue

Seventh Chakra: *Sahasrara* = Violet

Since each Chakra is represented by a different color and since there are so many ways to give color to your life, you can take care of each Chakra very easily. Chromotherapy is another method that you can use in total autonomy, you don't need any help to apply it, you just need to memorize the color associated with each Chakra. The enormous advantage of this method is that it takes no time at all, you only need to do is to choose carefully and consciously the colors that fill your life.

The three areas where you can use chromotherapy most effectively are your clothing, the food you eat, and your surroundings. For example, if you are working on the Sacral Chakra, you could wear a bright orange t-shirt, eat a juicy orange, and lay a bright orange bedspread on your bed.

Chromotherapy is a great way to work on multiple Chakras and also a quick way to intervene on a single one if you feel a momentary imbalance. When you get dressed in the morning you should choose at least one piece of clothing in the color of the Chakra you feel needs energizing. You should do the same with food, including in your food plan some food in harmony with the color of the Chakra to be harmonized.

As for the surrounding environment, since you can not change furniture too frequently, my advice is to create "spaces" dedicated to each one of the 7 colors in your house and in your working place. Then, you will only need to spend some time in a certain space when you feel the need to work on one color rather than another one. For example, you may need to spend 15 minutes on your "Red Space" because, at some point in your day, you don't feel as rooted in the moment as you should be.

One area that I recommend you devote a lot of attention to is your meditation corner. I have chosen to have in mine all the 7 colors represented in equivalent parts and then, when I feel the need for the predominance of the color of a certain Chakra, I temporarily add some object or decoration to make that color prevail over the others. Maybe I add a pillow, some flowers, a yoga mat, a stone, or a crystal that I then move and replace when I need to balance another Chakra associated with another color.

This last paragraph also introduced an important and interesting concept. Techniques for healing your Chakras often cross over, overlap, and support each other. For example, in your meditation corner in addition to the benefits of meditation, you will enjoy the benefits of chromotherapy, crystals, gemstones, and essential oils.

The care of the Chakras through colors is still a very effective technique, even alone, to find the balance of your Chakras and heal eventual blocks in the fluxing of energy.

Crystal Therapy

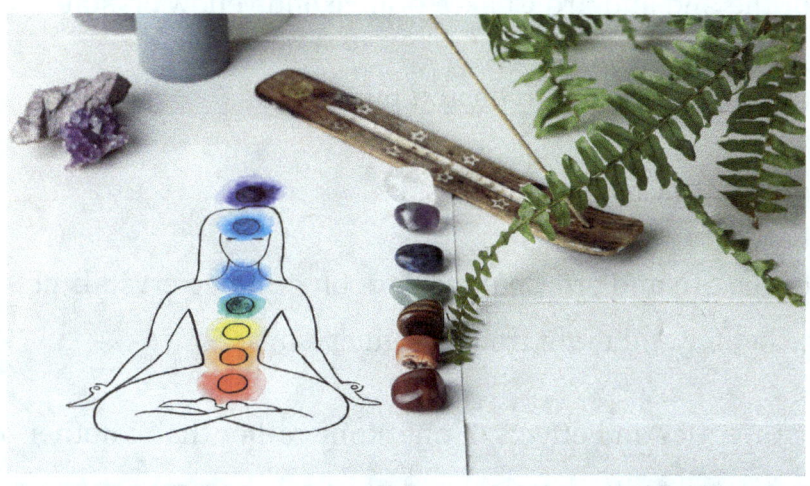

Crystal therapy allows us to use the power of stones, crystals, and minerals to restore the energetic balance of our Chakras, open them and unblock their energy flow if blocked. This method can be easily used in total independence.

To each specific Chakra corresponds a group of specific stones, as we have seen in the descriptive section of the 7 Chakras. The association between stone and Chakra occurs through color. The prevailing tonality of a Chakra is in resonance with the color of the stone. I summarized the color correspondence briefly below for your convenience. However, you can easily go back to the chapter titled "The 7 Main Chakras" to get more details on color correspondence, names of adequate gems, and crystals.

- For the 1st Chakra red, brown, and black crystals

- For the 2nd and 3rd Chakra orange and yellow crystals

- For the 4th Chakra green and pink crystals

- For the 5th Chakra blue crystals

- For the 6th and 7th Chakras dark blue-indigo crystals plus all the lighter and more transparent crystals.

The properties and effects of one stone rather than another one are subjected to its chemical and physical characteristics, as well as its color. For example, a piece of quartz and a piece of calcite of the same color will have different applications. The stones "preferred" by crystal therapy are, as you can deduce from the very name of this practice, quartz crystals. The crystal, in fact, has a high ability to absorb energy and activate the energy spectrum of a person. Crystals also stimulate intuition and awaken insight, helping us to nurture our spirituality, and supporting us in introspection, that is, helping us in our process of acquiring awareness.

There are many methods of using the power of stones to open, unlock and balance your Chakras. In the next pages, I will share with you the most important, useful, and easy to use.

Jewelry

There are jewelry pieces such as bracelets or necklaces that have different spherical stones strung in a sequence, just like the image below. They resonate with each one of the 7 Chakras.

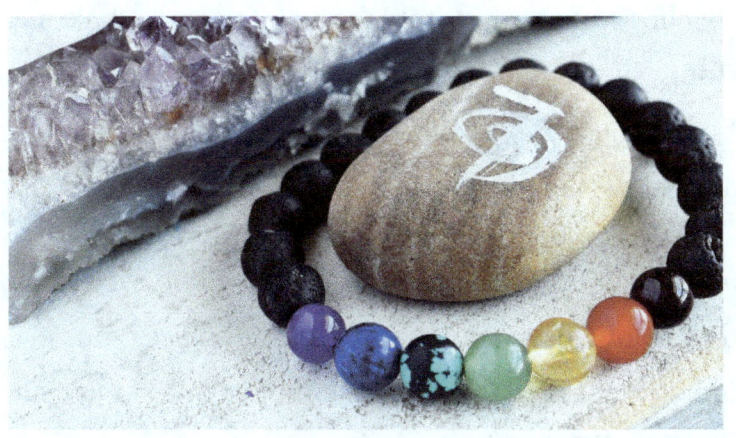

Wearing this jewelry regularly is a first step in harnessing the power of the stones to your advantage. This is nothing particularly expensive, it is jewelry made from hard stones and crystals, not precious stones. The shape of the stones is also not random, they are spherical to recall the shape and etymology of the Chakras. There are also variations of these jewels made with a single stone to work on a specific Chakra.

Corresponding Position Between Stone and Chakra

You'll need a set of stones, small enough in size, to perform this practice. You can easily find on sale in many shops ready-made kits containing a stone for each Chakra. I recommend, however, to go to a specialized store, if you have the opportunity, and personally choose a stone suitable to you for each Chakra. Take several stones in your hands, one at a time, and when you take the right one for you, you will feel it, because you will recognize the vibrations it is sending you.

When you have your 7 stones, using them will be very easy. You will need to lie down in a quiet and peaceful place, your meditation corner will be perfect if you have one set up. Then you will have to place each stone directly on your skin, in correspondence with the position in your body of the equivalent Chakra.

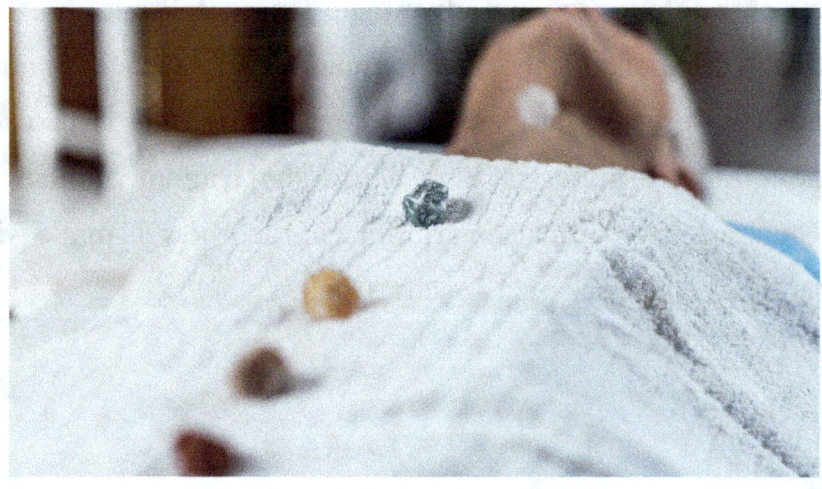

When the crystals are positioned you will have to close your eyes, concentrate on breathing, and visualize the energy of the stone placed on the first Chakra. The stone will do all the work, you just need to visualize for a few minutes, and then move on to the next stone and the next Chakra. You will have to proceed in order until you reach the Crown. You should lie there for at least 20 minutes, feeling the energy penetrating your body, and how the energy of each stone is channeled into its respective Chakra. In these 20 minutes, you should not move, you should not speak and you should let your thoughts be free to flow in your mind. Make sure that your breathing is steady and deep. Breathe through your nose. You should find this easy enough since you learned these basics in the chapter on meditation. Once you are done, take a few minutes before opening your eyes, during such time analyze how you feel, and enjoy the energy that is flowing through your body. Before you stand up again you will need to remove the stones. The removal should be in the opposite direction of placement, so you will need to start from the Crown and work your way down to the Root. (You may also choose to get help during the placement and removal if you have a trusted person who can help you, the important thing is that placement and removal are done in the correct order).

As in other practices, you can also practice this exercise on a single Chakra. You will use the single stone positioned on the Chakra concerned, in direct contact with your skin, and proceed with breathing and visualization, as explained in the previous lines.

In the following chart you will find an example of a stone for each Chakra and where to place it for a correct correspondence with its related Chakra:

Chakra	Crystal or Gem	Body Position
1º Chakra	Red Dispore	Groin
2º Chakra	Amber	Pelvis
3º Chakra	Citrin Quartz	Just above the navel
4º Chakra	Jade	Above the heart
5º Chakra	Aquamarine	On the throat
6º Chakra	Amethyst	On the forehead
7º Chakra	Hyaline Quartz	Press it on the top of your head, then place it on the surface where you are lying at the top of your head

Other Uses of Stones

There are many other options for using the energy and power of stones, gems, and crystals to your advantage. Since you can choose from a variety of sizes, there are so many uses to which they lend themselves.

For example, if you choose rather small pieces you could always carry one with you in your pocket and enjoy its energy constantly. Just reach into your pocket and squeeze your stone for an energy booster anytime you feel it's needed.

If you move frequently for work, you could keep one in your car to energize the environment in which you will be moving around. If you move by other means, you could put one in your bag or suitcase to carry the energy with you and feel its presence even when you are traveling.

As you can see, there are many ideas and, for sure, you will come up with others dictated by the very energy of the stones that will communicate with you. For example, I always keep one under the pillow I sleep with. I pick a different crystal every week and I change it on a color rotation.

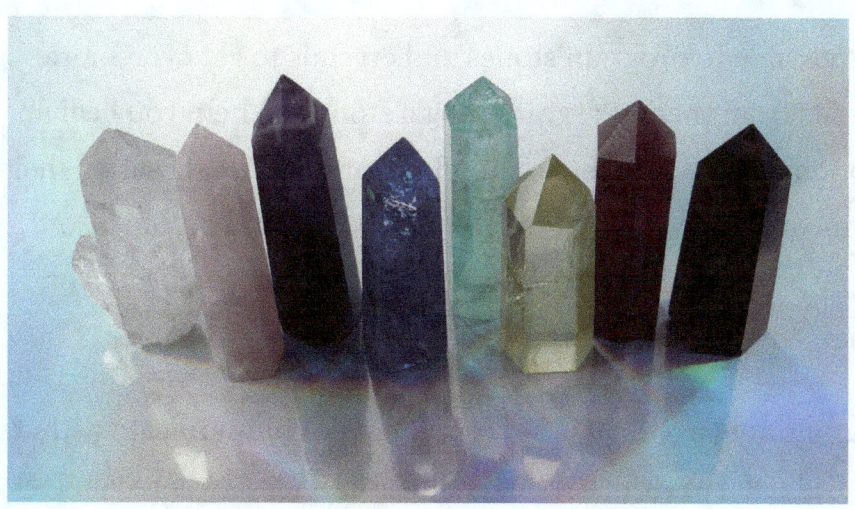

It is also useful to surround yourself with stones by using them to decorate your surroundings. For this option, it is usually better to choose larger stones. Place one for each Chakra at different points of the house so that their energy surrounds you. Having them around will make you feel better and you will find yourself walking around the house with a smile on your face. I recommend this decorative method in your meditation corner as well. Place a stone for each Chakra to decorate your corner, enrich the energy already present, and give more effectiveness to all the activities that you will do in that space. As I mentioned before, here are the various healing methods that intertwine with each other to give you greater results and an overall sensation of well-being.

Programming Your Stones

It is possible to program stones and crystals to get even more benefits from them. Programming a stone can help you heal an emotional wound, relieve an unpleasant physical sensation, help you meditate, or support you in a time of need. You can also simply program it to let you know if it needs to be purified or recharged with new energy.

Programming a crystal is very simple, just communicate with it. You will need to sit in a quiet and peaceful place where you feel comfortable, like your meditation corner, for example. You will have to close your eyes, enclose the stone inside your hand, feel it, and then start talking to it. The stone will hear you and, within a short time, you will receive your responses in the form of insights. Examples of stones' programming are, "Please, can you give me support today?"; "Please, can you tell me when you need to be purified or recharged?"; "Please, can you tell me what is the right choice to heal from my disappointment in love?". You can program your gems, stones, and crystals with this method for whatever need you might have.

Dialogue with your stones is very important and will make a difference in the results. You must put your heart into it and speak with intentionality. If you do it skeptically or just for the sake of doing it, it won't work. Listen to your heart and it will help you build an effective dialogue between you and your stone. Remember to choose the correct stone, choose one that corresponds to the Chakra that deals with the area of your request. For example, if your request is connected to emotions you need to pick a gem or a crystal in resonance with the Heart Chakra. If it is a request based on material things you need to pick a gemstone or a crystal in resonance with the Root Chakra.

Once you have programmed your stone, as your days go by, you will feel impulses, intuitions, and sensations that your stone will send you in response. For example, it will come to your mind to purify or recharge your stone, you will feel a sensation of support in the moment of need, or you will feel you must go to a certain place, where you will meet someone who, in time, will make you forget your disappointment of love.

Take a few minutes to program your stones and crystals. They will become your greatest allies in achieving mental, emotional, spiritual, and physical well-being. Trust me, you will feel like you own a real magical amulet.

Purifying Your Stones

Stones and crystals not only take energy from us, but also from our surroundings. This means that if you live in cities or highly populated places your crystals and stones will need to be cleansed from time to time of low frequency or unpleasant energies assimilated into your surroundings.

There are three main methods for purifying stones:

1. WATER: This first method is the simplest, but is ineffective on some particular stones. Use your dialogue with the stone to see if the cleaning is successful, or, if in doubt, use the third method which is the most effective. Simply place the stone under running water and, as you do so, visualize the unpleasant energy draining from the stone, and running away with the water.

2. WATER AND SALT: Again, this technique is not suitable for all stones because, although salt is a great purifier, it may damage some of the more polished or shiny stones. However, if you are certain that your stone is compatible with this method, simply soak it overnight in a glass of water and salt, then rinse it under running water the next morning. If in doubt about this method, I recommend using the third method, since it is the safest and most reliable.

3. INCENSE: This is the best and most effective method and, moreover, is good for all stones. Just light a natural incense and pass the stone in its smoke for about 30 seconds. As you do so, you should visualize the unpleasant energy that leaves your stone. You can also ask aloud as you perform the purification ritual, "Please cleanse this stone of any unpleasant energy, thank you!"

Just as with programming, the intentionality of the gesture is fundamental. Don't do it mechanically, just for the sake of doing it, but do it with the intention of purifying your crystals to get the maximum benefit from them. This will make a huge difference to the effectiveness of your purification rituals.

Recharging Your Stones

Recharging your stones periodically with beneficial energy is of fundamental importance because they will then share this energy with you.

There are three main methods for recharging stones and crystals with beneficial energy:

1. THE SUN: The best sunlight to energize your stones is at dawn. Expose the stones in a place where they can get direct sunlight in the early morning. A couple of hours will be sufficient. Ideally, this should be from 6 to 8 a.m., in winter even up to 9 a.m. Remember to remove your stones and crystals from the sun when the light is particularly intense, to avoid damaging them. A timer or an alarm clock will be useful as a reminder.

2. THE MOON: To energize your stones through the moonlight, you'll need a full moon night. Simply display your stones and crystals somewhere in the house near a window where they can enjoy the benefits of the full moon's light. You will need to remove the stones from where you placed them before sunrise before the sunlight hits them in full.

3. THE EARTH: To use the earth's energy on your stones, trees are perfect, but a potted plant will also do. You will need to place the stones on the earth at the foot of the tree or in the pot of your plant. If the sun is beating down at the location you've chosen, you'll need to place your stones in a small hole dug in the earth, and cover them. You can wrap them in a bit of paper to prevent them from getting dirty. It will only take a few hours to energize your stones with soil, but you can also leave them for a few days in total safety.

Essential Oils Therapy

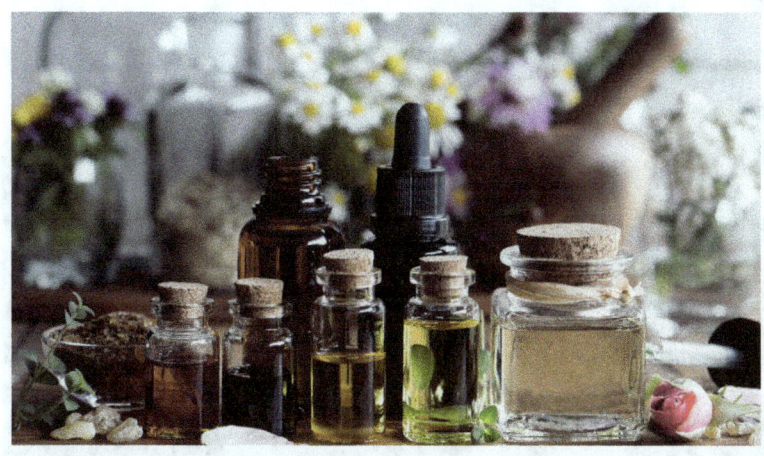

When I discussed the characteristics of every single Chakra, I also described the scents connected to each of them. The scents that we associate with each Chakra are essential oils from plants that can be used in many simple ways to have results similar to chromotherapy and crystal therapy.

Each essential oil has its own Chakra and there are many options for using these oils. The simplest method is to use a "burner" that will spread the chosen fragrance throughout your home or other surroundings. This practice is called aromatherapy. Just pour a few drops of oil into the water of your burner, turn on the flame underneath, and immediately the fragrance will begin to spread in the air (the method described is that of a classic burner, but there are many varieties and each comes with instructions if should follow carefully).

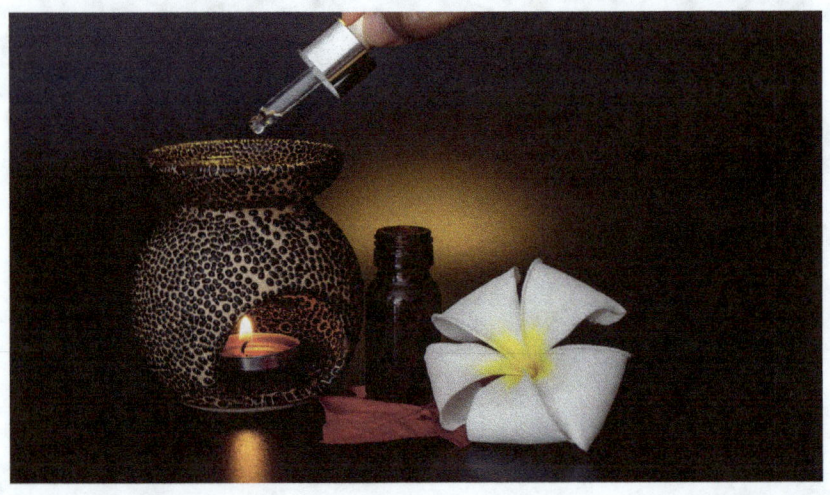

This method is great to practice in your meditation corner because it can easily be combined with other healing techniques to make them even more effective. For example, if you are meditating for a particular Chakra, sprinkling the aroma of the oil associated with it will make your meditation much deeper and more effective.

Another use of essential oils extremely effective to unlock and balance your Chakras is to use them during massages directly on your skin. Essential oils facilitate the massage by making your hands glide better. To perform the massage you must mix a few drops of the essential oil chosen to treat your Chakra with a neutral oil specifically for massage (for example, jojoba oil). It is important to treat only one Chakra at a time with this method, making the massage with extreme delicacy, and dedicating to the massage all the time necessary to open, unblock the energy, and put it back into circulation.

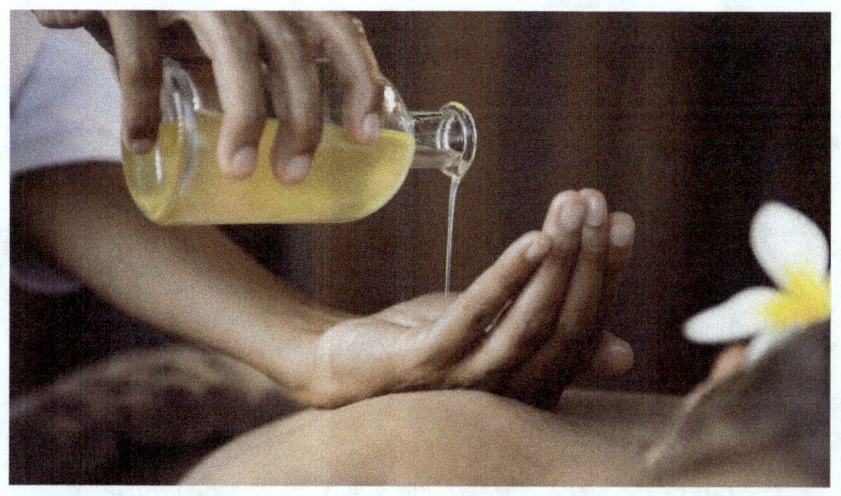

In one of the previous paragraphs, you learned how and which areas to massage to open, unblock, and balance a Chakra. By combining the massage with the essential oil corresponding to that Chakra, you can double the effectiveness of your massage, and the energy released. If you like, without exaggerating, you can also diffuse in the environment the same fragrance you are using for the massage, involving more senses in the unlocking and balancing of your energies.

Let's see together the associations between Chakra, massage, and essential oil, in one of the usual practical summarizing charts:

Chakra	Areas to Massage	Essential Oils
1° Chakra	Buttocks, legs, and feet	Sandalwood, patchouli, and cypress
2° Chakra	Below the navel, the hips, and the base of the back	Jasmine, pine, and ylang-ylang
3° Chakra	Abdomen and stomach	Mint, black pepper, and cloves
4° Chakra	Chest and shoulders	Rose, sweet orange, and lemon balm
5° Chakra	The base of the neck and neck	Eucalyptus, chamomile, and verbena
6° Chakra	Face	Neroli, mint, and thyme
7° Chakra	Head and scalp	Olibanum, jasmine, and sandalwood

You will have noticed that some oils are effective for more than one Chakra according to the different characteristics that they possess. When you choose an oil to use always make sure to pick the scent you prefer, and with which you feel comfortable. This is the most effective way to obtain the best result. In fact, if you use an oil whose smell you don't truly like, you will end up with headaches and discomfort.

The connection between essential oils and Chakra, therefore, allows you to easily restore the balance of a Chakra at the moment in which this balance should fail. It also allows you to maintain a correct and constant flow of energy, take care of yourself, and maintain your physical, mental, spiritual, and emotional well-being.

You can apply this great method in total independence, fully enjoying its powerful results. There is one factor, however, that you must pay attention to when using essential oils to help your Chakras. It is the quality of the oils. Many oils on the market, especially the cheaper ones, are not pure and are not good for your Chakra healing journey. You must always make sure to buy pure oils. It is not difficult to find them, they are now widespread, and you can find them more or less everywhere. Before making your purchase be sure to carefully read the label where it is indicated the composition of the oil, to avoid wrong purchases. Also try to buy from stores that have testers, especially in the beginning. This will help you figure out if a fragrance is right for you and will prevent you from spending money unnecessarily. Since quality oils are a little more expensive than impure ones, it's best to buy something you're sure you'll use.

Before we move on to the benefits chapter, I'd like to close this section with one last piece of advice: only use one oil to start with. I know you may want to use this method right away to clear more than one Chakra and you are eager to try different oils but it is important to start slowly. You must try a single oil for a few days to understand how you and your body react to the fragrance and to this practice. If all goes well, you can begin to expand your selection of fragrances to use and continue to expand it over time.

The Power of Chakras: Benefits of Healthy Chakras on Physical, Mental, Emotional, and Spiritual Levels

Having open, healthy Chakras, free from blockages and with a balanced energy flow will allow you to enjoy a state of pleasant health on a mental, emotional, spiritual, and physical level. I think at this point in the book this concept is already clear to you. However, I would like to address in detail some of the greatest benefits that you will enjoy so that they can serve as a spur to begin immediately your path of analysis, healing, and maintenance of your Chakras.

Chakras' care is what we call holistic medicine. Holistic medicine takes care of the physical, mental, spiritual, and emotional aspects of a person at the same time; as opposed to traditional medicine which only treats one at a time according to the symptoms. If you suffer from any disease or have any health problems, you should always continue to take care of your body according to the medical prescription you get from your doctor. Studying and healing your Chakras can be a positive support to whatever path of healing and care you are following because it will take care of your emotions, your spiritual side, and your mental side, making the care of your body more efficient. This book is not intended in any way to replace medicine, but only to help you feel better, teaching you how to prevent discomfort, take care of your body, and always work in support of your well-being, through all the benefits that the energy of the Chakras can give you when it flows properly in your body.

Let's see together the main benefits.

You'll Feel More Positive

One of the first changes you will notice after working on your Chakras and balancing them is that you will feel more positive. When all the Chakras are open, healthy, and balanced, you are in a state of physical, mental, spiritual, and emotional well-being. This new feeling of overall wellness allows you to see everything in a new, more positive light. You will easily see the positive side of things. You'll understand people and their behavior better, so you won't distress yourself by seeing their actions as an attack on you. You'll be aware that sometimes things don't go the way you want them to but that soon the wheel will turn on your side. You will see this and much more. You will see your world and your reality with new eyes. You will finally see the beauty of the world around you.

You'll Be Less Sad

Having the Chakras in balance eliminates the sense of sadness and helps us to know how to deal with it when it arises due to a negative circumstance such as for example, the loss of a loved one.

When the Chakra energy flows correctly and without blockages, your vision of the world is so clear that you can understand that everything that happens to you happens for a specific reason. This awareness makes you live more positively, as I pointed out at the beginning of this chapter, and this removes the sense of sadness.

Moreover, when your Chakras are healthy and balanced, you are not blocked by stress or unmanageable, and out-of-control emotions, so you are not in danger of being overwhelmed by unmotivated sadness.

If at this moment, you are experiencing a sense of sadness because of a particular event in your life or for no reason, you need to work on the Fourth, Sixth and Seventh Chakras. The Sixth, and Seventh Chakras are particularly important in this circumstance because they influence your spiritual sphere and the relationship with a higher power that allows you to accept and deal with events that can bring sadness.

You'll Manage Anger Better

If each Chakra is well balanced, you will very rarely get angry, and if you do, it will be very easy to manage.

The regular practice of Chakra meditation and Yoga sessions will help you, more than any other exercise, to enjoy this benefit.

It is important to be free of the ballast of anger because it influences several negative factors in our lives. If you act out of anger and in anger, you will end up with personal, professional, and health problems.

The fundamental Chakra to focus on if you have problems controlling and eliminating anger from your life is the Fourth, the Heart Chakra. You will have to concentrate on your exercises to get its perfect balance. The Fourth Chakra influences emotions and its balance allows us not to be overwhelmed by them, or let them get out of control. In this way, you will be able to manage and eliminate anger.

You'll Sleep Better

The importance of sleep concerning a person's health has been underestimated for too long and it is only in recent years that studies on the subject are emphasizing its importance.

Lack of sleep or poor quality sleep negatively affects the state of our body, mind, and spirit. You've probably had a bad night's sleep and got up in the morning in a bad mood, with little mental clarity, a little sore, constantly hungry, and wanting to eat junk food. Think about what damage a stressful situation of the type just described can cause in your life, especially if it is repeated more or less frequently.

You'll be down in the dumps, in a bad mood, and maybe a little depressed. All the junk food will give you stomach problems and, probably, your skin will show unwelcome pimples. The lack of mental clarity will lead you, in the long run, to make poor choices and poorly reasoned, with all the precipitation of events that this can cause. From this situation of mental, physical, and emotional stress, your immune system comes out extremely tested, with all the consequences that this entails.

Fortunately, when Chakras' energy flows properly through your body and puts it in a state of total well-being, the quality and quantity of your sleep are no longer an issue. You'll sleep well for as long as your body needs. You will know this for sure, both because of the feeling of wellness you will experience, and because by following the exercises in this book you will have learned to communicate with your body, and listen to its messages.

The use of Chakras' meditation in any of its forms helps a lot to ensure the quality of your sleep. It puts you in such a state of well-being that your body will not find blocks or obstacles to falling asleep. In addition, meditation helps you to better dialogue with your body, and you will receive useful messages, in case you need to intervene in some way to further improve your sleep (That's why I have often repeated the importance of the last step of meditation, which is to analyze how you feel, before opening your eyes again).

Usually, it is the First, Third, and Fourth Chakras that influence sleep. If you find that the quality of your sleep is not adequate or you feel that you are not getting enough sleep, you could dedicate your Chakras' meditation in turn to these three specific Chakras, to rebalance their state of health. Alternatively, you can focus on one particular Chakra by identifying which one is causing the problem. The first Chakra affects sleep in general and its quality. If, however, you feel you don't want to sleep, the cause may be the Third Chakra. If instead, you feel very tired even at a mental level, but you can't sleep at all, the fault is of the Fourth Chakra.

Linked to this topic is the discussion about dreams. If your sleep problems are in some way related to dreams, then you must work on the Sixth Chakra, because the problem comes from the unconscious and it is the Sixth Chakra that deals with it. Take care of your Chakras to sleep well.

Only thanks to healthy and balanced Chakras will you sleep better and enjoy the benefits of better sleep, avoiding the discomfort, and stress that inadequate sleep causes in a person's life.

You'll Be Less Stressed

Doing exercises to maintain Chakra balance and practicing Chakra meditation regularly will help you gradually eliminate stress from your life.

Living a stress-free life brings a whole host of benefits, which you're probably familiar with, but are worth remembering.

First of all, as we mentioned earlier, being stress-free allows you to rest better, and see life in a more positive light. Stress often brings with it a sense of anxiety, a feeling of emotional blockage, and is also a real obstruction to achieving your goals, and what you want to achieve in life. Without it, you will be calmer, more emotionally balanced, and finally ready to get everything you want out of life.

So, practice daily all the methods you have learned in this book to keep your Chakras balanced and enjoy the benefits of a stress-free life.

You'll Manage Depression Better

When your Chakras are aligned and functioning well you will feel in control of your life and emotions, free from stress, energetic, bubbly, and full of zest for life.

When these elements are lacking in your life then you begin to feel a sense of depression. Depression comes from a feeling of lack of control over your life and your emotions. This sense of lack of control causes energy loss, apathy, weakness, and stress.

To manage the onset of a sense of depression you will need to focus your exercises on the First, Third, and Seventh Chakras. In a couple of weeks, you will begin to feel the first benefits. You will feel the energy that begins to increase, you will want to move and do physical activity. Stress will slowly recede from your life along with depression.

By keeping your Chakras in good health and perfect balance over time, you will be in continuous control of your life and these unpleasant feelings will become increasingly rare, even disappearing with the constancy in taking care of yourself.

You'll Have Healthier Relationships with People

When your Chakras are working at their best, you will feel at ease with people, stable balanced in their presence, and it will be easy to accept novelty and change in your relationships with them. You will be able to build healthy relationships with those around you without problems, you will know to whom to give your trust without fear, and you won't be overwhelmed by what you feel for those people.

Every relationship in a person's life touches so many points that all the Chakras end up being involved. Only the complete balance between all 7 Chakras allows us to live our relationships with others in the best way. A healthy relationship with others is fundamental to living our lives well. On the contrary, an unhealthy relationship brings with it negative energies along with all the consequences that negative energies cause in us, and in our lives.

By the term "relationship with others", I mean a relationship with a family member, a friend, or a partner. When we feel unstable with someone or we just can't trust even those who are reliable in a proven way, then we need to balance the First Chakra.

When the problems are in sexual or emotional relationships where we are too rigid and inflexible, then we need to balance the Second Chakra.

If emotions and confidence are unstable and, therefore, we become aggressive towards others then we need to balance the Third Chakra.

If we don't realize that we are loved and we can't feel the right emotions then we need to balance the Fourth Chakra.

If we fail to communicate with friends, family, or partners then we need to balance the Fifth Chakra.

If we cannot overcome differences of opinion, petty disputes, and disagreements with people around us then we need to balance the Sixth Chakra.

If we cannot think clearly and objectively and we act angrily when interacting with a person, perhaps excluding that person completely from our lives then we need to balance the Seventh Chakra.

As you can easily see by yourself, only a perfect balance of all 7 Chakras can allow you to have healthy and balanced relationships with people, and enjoy the benefits that this state brings. So, make sure to take care of your energy doors regularly to enjoy all the benefits that this balance can bring into your life.

You'll Be More Passionate

To fully enjoy life, it is important to live all its aspects with passion and appreciate all it has to offer.

By keeping your Chakras healthy and balanced with daily exercises and meditation, you will be able to live all aspects of your life with passion, such as your work, your family, your hobbies, and of course your relationship with your partner.

When your Chakras are well balanced you will see the world around you from a better perspective and it will be easier to enjoy what it has to offer. You will feel connected to this wonderful world, you will feel part of it, and ready for all the beautiful things it has in store for you. All of this will make you live your daily activities and your sex life with passion.

There is a close connection between the passion you put into your daily activities and the passion you experience in your bedroom. If you are going through a cold spell in sexual passion, take a look at your life, and, almost certainly, you will notice that you lack passion in a lot of other areas.

Get your Chakra energy flowing smoothly and balanced to enjoy the passion you deserve in all areas of your life.

You'll Achieve Your Goals

When your Chakras are healthy and their energy flows balanced, it is easier to get results, improve your performance, and achieve your goals. This happens because the state of well-being that we experience allows us to perform to the best of our abilities, without anything blocking, or hindering us. We feel so well that everything becomes easy to achieve.

There is no stress to hinder us, so we sleep well and feel good. This wellness allows us to have excellent performance in whatever area we are interested in, it allows us to build healthy, balanced, and positive relationships with the people we want in our lives. In addition, since we feel free from blocks, our self-confidence is very high, and this is an essential element to achieving personal success.

You'll Strengthen Your Body and Set in Motion a Prevention Mechanism

Our minds and our emotions act directly on our bodies. As I have repeatedly pointed out in this book, by taking care of your energy points, you will ensure mental, spiritual, and emotional health that will have beneficial consequences on your body and your physical health.

If you have never taken care of your Chakras until now, probably your emotional, mental, and spiritual conditions have somehow afflicted your body as well. You will see things change very fast when you become familiar with the DIY techniques to take care of yourself I shared with you in the previous chapter.

If, for example, you live in a constant situation of mental and emotional stress, you may be very overweight, always have a runny nose, a cold, a headache, or a constant sense of fatigue even when you do little or nothing. This happens because you sleep badly, eat poorly, waste energy because you can't think straight, and so on. I think you know very well what I'm talking about.

When your Chakras are open, healthy, functioning, and balanced, you experience such a positive emotional, spiritual, and mental condition that you lessen the negative repercussions on your body until they go away.

It has been scientifically proven that stress and depression damage your immune system, making you easy prey to bacteria and viruses that cause flues and colds, but also other diseases. The state of well-being you find yourself in when your Chakras are balanced, on the other hand, increases and strengthens the health of your immune system because you eliminate the damage caused by stress and depression in your life.

In short, by taking care of your Chakras with constancy you will set in motion a mechanism of prevention that will allow you to significantly raise the quality of your life. With your Chakras open and balanced you can take care of yourself by living a healthy life on a physical, mental, emotional, and spiritual level.

Conclusion

We have come to the end of our journey together and I would like to thank you for following me this far. Before letting you go, I would like to draw the conclusions from what we have said so far and leave you with some final advice and considerations.

In the first part of the book, you've learned the basics about the characteristics of each Chakra. At this point, you are perfectly able to analyze yourself physically, mentally, emotionally, and spiritually to understand where to begin your journey to open, unlock, and balance your Chakras. With the notions I have shared with you, you are able to associate your "symptoms" to the corresponding Chakra, and make your own "diagnosis". Now that you know which Chakra needs your attention, you can use all the DIY techniques shown in the second part of this book to open, heal, unblock, and balance it.

There isn't a Chakra more important than another one. To choose wisely the one to prioritize, you simply need to analyze your situation, how are you feeling now, and start from the areas that cause you more suffering and discomfort.

If you can not find a precise starting point, my advice is to start doing exercises for unlocking and rebalancing all the 7 Chakras, addressing them in order, from the lowest to the highest. The most efficient exercise that I recommend to you at this stage of confusion is "The 7 Chakras' meditation" which will allow you to see things in a clearer light. This technique will also give you the best results in the shortest time on all levels of your being: physical, mental, spiritual, and emotional.

Another piece of advice I would like to share with you is to create a Chakra routine for yourself. I used this method myself when I started to approach this discipline, and it helped me a lot. We, humans, are very habitual beings, and doing something new is always a bit complicated, especially at the beginning when we are not yet used to it. Building a routine and starting to practice it will help you to implement Chakra healing in your daily life.

Let me explain. Choose the practices that best suit you among those I have illustrated and begin to incorporate them into your daily routine, giving them specific spaces. My main problem was that I tended to forget new things, so I used sticky notes as reminders. Let me give you an example. I had arranged my house so that each different area was dedicated to a color, the prevalence of one color in a specific area of the house helped the corresponding Chakra. Also, I had taped on my closet and in the kitchen a chart where I assigned a color to each day of the week, and that day I dedicated clothing and food portions to that color. This was my method for using color therapy.

I had a list of 7 affirmations, one for each Chakra, that I kept taped to my bathroom mirror as a reminder to repeat them in the morning as soon as I woke up, and at night before I went to bed, so I wouldn't forget to use positive affirmations to balance my Chakras.

I had also created my own meditation corner at home, furnishing it with semiprecious stones and essence burners, as well as colorful rugs and fabrics. I had set reminders on my phone, at times when I was sure to be home, to remind me of meditation time, rather than massage, or stone therapy time.

It may seem a bit rigid and schematic at first, but it is the best method to develop the habit of taking care of your Chakras. In 3 or 4 weeks the habit will begin to consolidate and it will become spontaneous for you to perform various actions for your daily well-being. From that moment on, you will realize that the bar for the quality of your life will be raised a little higher every day, and you will probably no longer need sticky notes and reminders because taking care of yourself will become spontaneous.

Once you have unlocked your Chakras, don't let them get stuck again. Pay attention to your body's signals and the emotional, mental, and spiritual messages you receive in the form of intuitions. They will tell you immediately if a particular Chakra is about to get blocked, close, or get out of balance, and you can immediately intervene on it with one or more of the methods you have learned in this book.

My advice is to practice your Chakra routine daily, or at least as regularly as possible according to your schedule, to keep stable the balance you have obtained. This will prevent most of the future blocks and imbalances from occurring and keep you and your Chakras in a state of health and wellness.

Now we have truly come to the time of farewells.

I hope I have helped you in some way with my experience. I hope you have enjoyed this journey together and that it has been as enjoyable for you as it has been for me to accompany you in the discovery of the energy points of your body. Thanks for being with me and have a nice life

Namasté

Anja

Mind, Body, and Spirit Masterclass

www.ingramcontent.com/pod-product-compliance
Lightning Source LLC
Chambersburg PA
CBHW070640120526
44590CB00013BA/799